INTRODUCTION

Mast Cell Activation Syndrome (MCAS) is a complex and often underdiagnosed medical condition characterized by the aberrant activation of mast cells throughout the body. Mast cells, a type of immune cell, play a vital role in the body's defense against pathogens and in maintaining tissue homeostasis. However, in individuals with MCAS, these mast cells become hyperresponsive, releasing excessive mediators, such as histamine, prostaglandins, and cytokines. This uncontrolled release of mediators can lead to many symptoms that affect multiple organ systems, including the skin, gastrointestinal tract, respiratory system, and cardiovascular system.

The clinical presentation of MCAS is diverse, making diagnosis challenging. Symptoms can range from skin rashes, abdominal pain, and nausea to headaches, fatigue, and cardiovascular issues. Due to its wide-ranging and often nonspecific symptoms, MCAS is frequently misdiagnosed or overlooked, delaying appropriate management.

In recent years, the role of diet in managing MCAS has gained attention as part of a holistic approach to symptom control. While no one-size-fits-all dietary solution exists for individuals with MCAS, certain nutritional modifications may help alleviate symptoms and improve quality of life.

One dietary consideration in managing MCAS is the adoption of a histamine-restricted diet. Histamine, a key mediator released by activated mast cells, can trigger or exacerbate symptoms in some individuals. Foods high in histamine, such as aged cheeses, fermented products, and certain fruits and vegetables, may be restricted to minimize symptom occurrence.

Additionally, an individualized approach to identifying trigger foods is crucial. Keeping a detailed food diary and working closely with healthcare professionals, including allergists and registered dietitians, can help pinpoint specific dietary triggers unique to each person. This personalized approach allows for developing a tailored dietary plan that addresses the particular needs and sensitivities of the individual with MCAS.

Furthermore, an anti-inflammatory diet rich in fruits, vegetables, whole grains, and omega-3 fatty acids may be beneficial for some individuals with MCAS. This approach aims to reduce overall inflammation in the body, potentially mitigating the hyperactivity of mast cells and the resulting symptomatology.

CHAPTER ONE

Understanding Mast Cell Activation Syndrome (MCAS)

Mast Cell Activation Syndrome (MCAS) is a complex and often underdiagnosed medical condition characterized by an abnormal and excessive activation of mast cells, a type of immune cell in various body tissues. These mast cells play a crucial role in the immune system, serving as critical responders to allergic reactions and contributing to the regulation of inflammatory processes.

In individuals with MCAS, mast cells become hyperresponsive, releasing an array of mediators such as histamine, prostaglandins, and cytokines. This uncontrolled release of mediators can result in a wide range of symptoms, affecting multiple organ systems and giving rise to a diverse clinical presentation.

MAST CELL ACTIVATION SYNDROME (MCAS) SYMPTOMS

Mast Cell Activation Syndrome (MCAS) is characterized by a broad spectrum of symptoms that can affect various organ systems throughout the body. The diverse and often unpredictable nature of these symptoms poses challenges in both diagnosis and management. The following are common symptoms associated with MCAS:

1. Skin Symptoms:
    a. Hives (Urticaria): Raised, itchy welts on the skin that can appear suddenly and vary in size.
    b. Itching (Pruritus): Persistent or episodic itching, often without visible rash.
    c. Flushing: Sudden redness or warmth of the skin, sometimes accompanied by a sensation of heat.
2. Respiratory Symptoms:
    a. Wheezing: A high-pitched whistling sound produced during breathing indicates airway constriction.

    b. Shortness of Breath: Difficulty breathing, often accompanied by a feeling of tightness in the chest.

3. Gastrointestinal Symptoms:

    a. Abdominal Pain: Discomfort or pain in the abdominal region can vary in intensity and duration.

    b. Diarrhea: Frequent, loose, or watery stools.

    c. Nausea: A sensation of discomfort in the stomach, sometimes leading to the urge to vomit.

4. Cardiovascular Symptoms:

    a. Rapid Heart Rate (Tachycardia): An elevated heart rate, which palpitations may accompany.

    b. Low Blood Pressure (Hypotension): A drop in blood pressure, potentially leading to dizziness or fainting.

5. Neurological Symptoms:

    a. Headaches: Persistent or recurrent headaches, which can vary in intensity and duration.

    b. Brain Fog: Cognitive impairment characterized by difficulties with concentration, memory, and mental clarity.

    c. Dizziness: A feeling of lightheadedness or unsteadiness.

6. Musculoskeletal Symptoms:

    a. Joint Pain: Discomfort or pain in the joints, resembling symptoms of arthritis.

b. Muscle Pain: Aching or soreness in the muscles, often accompanied by fatigue.

CAUSES AND TRIGGERS OF MAST CELL ACTIVATION

The causes and triggers of mast cell activation are diverse, encompassing a combination of genetic factors, environmental influences, and various stressors. Understanding these factors is crucial for managing and mitigating the symptoms associated with MCAS.

1. Genetic Factors:
   a. Inherited Predisposition: There is evidence to suggest a genetic component in MCAS, with some individuals having a genetic predisposition to mast cell abnormalities. Specific gene mutations or variations may contribute to the hyperresponsiveness of mast cells.
2. Environmental Triggers:
   a. Allergens: Exposure to allergens, such as pollen, pet dander, and mold, can trigger mast cell activation in susceptible individuals.
   b. Environmental Toxins: Certain environmental toxins, pollutants, and

chemicals may contribute to mast cell activation. Sensitivity to these substances can vary among individuals.

3. Stress and Emotional Factors:
    a. Psychological Stress: Emotional stress, anxiety, and other psychological factors can trigger mast cell activation. Stress may act as a modulator, exacerbating symptoms in individuals with MCAS.
    b. Physical Stress: Intense physical exertion, illness, or surgery can also act as stressors that trigger mast cell activation.

4. Common Triggers:
    a. Foods: Certain foods are known to trigger mast cell activation, especially those high in histamine or other biogenic amines. Examples include fermented foods, aged cheeses, tomatoes, and certain fruits.
    b. Medications: Some medications, such as nonsteroidal anti-inflammatory drugs (NSAIDs), certain antibiotics, and muscle relaxants, can trigger mast cell activation in susceptible individuals.
    c. Insect Stings and Bites: Venom from insect stings or bites, such as those from bees, wasps, or ants, can induce a strong mast cell response in individuals with MCAS.
    d. Temperature Changes: Extreme temperatures, both hot and cold, can be triggers for mast cell activation in some

individuals.

DIAGNOSIS OF MAST CELL ACTIVATION SYNDROME (MCAS)

Diagnosing Mast Cell Activation Syndrome (MCAS) is a complex process involving clinical evaluation, medical history, laboratory tests, and the careful exclusion of other potential conditions. Due to the broad and diverse range of symptoms associated with MCAS, a thorough and systematic approach is essential.

1. Clinical Evaluation and Medical History:
    a. Symptom Assessment: A comprehensive evaluation of the patient's symptoms is a crucial starting point. Symptoms associated with MCAS can affect various organ systems, including the skin, respiratory, gastrointestinal, cardiovascular, neurological, and musculoskeletal systems.
    b. Medical History: Gathering a detailed medical history, including information about the onset, duration, and

progression of symptoms, as well as any potential triggers or exacerbating factors, is essential for understanding the patient's clinical picture.

2. Laboratory Tests for Mast Cell Mediators:

   a. Serum Tryptase Levels: Tryptase is a crucial mediator activated mast cell release. Serum tryptase levels are often measured to assess baseline mast cell activity. However, normal tryptase levels do not rule out MCAS, as elevations may not always be present during episodes of activation.

   b. Urinary N-Methylhistamine: Elevated levels of urinary N-methylhistamine, a metabolite of histamine, may indicate increased mast cell activity. This test can provide additional information on histamine release.

3. Provocation Testing and Challenges:

   a. Provocative Testing: In some cases, provocation testing may be employed to induce mast cell activation under controlled conditions. This can include the administration of specific triggers, such as medications or foods while monitoring for symptomatic responses.

   b. Oral Food Challenges: Controlled introduction of suspected trigger foods in a clinical setting can help identify specific dietary triggers.

4. Differential Diagnosis and Ruling Out Other Conditions:

a. Allergic and Immunologic Conditions: Allergic disorders, autoimmune diseases, and other immunologic conditions may present with symptoms similar to those of MCAS. A thorough evaluation is necessary to differentiate between these conditions.

b. Infectious Diseases: Certain infections can mimic the symptoms of MCAS. A careful assessment and appropriate testing help rule out infectious causes.

c. Endocrine Disorders: Conditions such as thyroid disorders and adrenal insufficiency can present with symptoms overlapping those of MCAS, necessitating evaluation of endocrine function.

TREATMENT APPROACHES FOR MCAS

The management of Mast Cell Activation Syndrome (MCAS) involves a multifaceted approach aimed at stabilizing mast cells, alleviating symptoms, and improving the overall quality of life for affected individuals. Treatment strategies often include a combination of medications, symptomatic relief measures, lifestyle modifications, and, in some cases, immunotherapy.

1. Medications to Stabilize Mast Cells:
   a. Antihistamines: These drugs, such as cetirizine, fexofenadine, and loratadine, can help block the effects of histamine released by mast cells. Antihistamines are often a first-line treatment for managing symptoms like itching, hives, and nasal congestion.
   b. Mast Cell Stabilizers: Medications like cromolyn sodium work by stabilizing mast cells and preventing the release of inflammatory mediators. These may be used to manage symptoms in some

cases.

2. Symptomatic Relief and Management of Specific Symptoms:

   a. Epinephrine (EpiPen): For individuals with a history of severe anaphylactic reactions triggered by MCAS, carrying an epinephrine auto-injector is often recommended to provide rapid relief in case of emergencies.

   b. Gastrointestinal Medications: Proton pump inhibitors (PPIs) or H2 blockers may be prescribed to manage symptoms such as acid reflux and abdominal pain.

   c. Analgesics: Pain relievers like acetaminophen may be recommended to manage musculoskeletal symptoms.

3. Lifestyle Modifications:

   a. Dietary Changes: Identifying and avoiding trigger foods, which can vary from person to person, is crucial to managing MCAS. Following a low-histamine diet and keeping a food diary can aid in pinpointing specific triggers.

   b. Stress Management: Stress can exacerbate symptoms in individuals with MCAS. Stress reduction techniques, such as mindfulness, meditation, and relaxation exercises, may be beneficial.

   c. Environmental Control: Minimizing exposure to environmental triggers, such as allergens and toxins, can help reduce the likelihood of mast cell activation.

4. Immunotherapy in Some Cases:
    a. Desensitization: In specific situations, allergen immunotherapy (allergy shots) may be considered to desensitize the immune system and reduce hypersensitivity reactions.
    b. Monoclonal Antibodies: Emerging therapies involve the use of monoclonal antibodies that target specific receptors involved in mast cell activation. Research in this area is ongoing and represents a potential avenue for future treatment options.

LIFESTYLE MODIFICATIONS IN MCAS MANAGEMENT

Lifestyle modifications play a crucial role in the management of Mast Cell Activation Syndrome (MCAS), complementing medical interventions and dietary adjustments. By incorporating specific lifestyle changes, individuals with MCAS can enhance their overall well-being and minimize the impact of mast cell activation on their daily lives.

1. Stress Management Techniques:
    a. Mindfulness and Meditation: Stress is a well-recognized trigger for mast cell activation. Mindfulness practices, such as meditation and deep breathing exercises, can help manage stress levels and promote relaxation.
    b. Yoga and Tai Chi: These gentle forms of exercise combine movement, breath control, and meditation, offering both physical and mental benefits. They may contribute to stress reduction and

improve overall resilience.

2. Identification and Avoidance of Triggers:
   a. Environmental Triggers: Beyond dietary considerations, individuals with MCAS often have specific environmental triggers. Identifying and avoiding these triggers, which may include allergens, pollutants, or certain chemicals, is essential for symptom management.
   b. Personalized Trigger Management: Keeping a detailed diary to track daily activities, symptoms, and potential triggers helps individuals identify patterns and make informed decisions about lifestyle modifications. This personalized approach allows for better control of symptom triggers.
3. Exercise and its Role in Symptom Management:
   a. Moderate Exercise: Engaging in regular, moderate exercise can have positive effects on overall health and may contribute to symptom management. However, it's essential to tailor exercise routines to individual capabilities and energy levels.
   b. Adapted Activities: Low-impact exercises, such as walking, swimming, or gentle stretching, can be well-tolerated by many individuals with MCAS. The goal is to find activities that promote fitness without exacerbating symptoms.
4. Sleep Hygiene Considerations:

a. Establishing a Routine: Consistent sleep patterns and a regular sleep-wake cycle contribute to improved sleep quality. Establishing a bedtime routine and maintaining a consistent sleep schedule can be beneficial.

b. Creating a Restful Environment: Minimizing environmental factors that may disrupt sleep, such as excessive light and noise, can enhance the quality of sleep for individuals with MCAS.

c. Addressing Sleep Disorders: Identifying and managing sleep disorders, such as insomnia or sleep apnea, is crucial. Poor sleep can exacerbate symptoms and impact overall well-being.

5. Hydration and Nutrition:

a. Adequate Hydration: Staying well-hydrated is essential for flushing out toxins and potentially reducing the concentration of mast cell mediators. Individuals with MCAS should maintain sufficient fluid intake.

b. Balanced Nutrition: A well-balanced diet that meets nutritional needs is crucial for overall health. This includes incorporating a variety of nutrient-dense foods and addressing any specific dietary restrictions based on individual triggers.

THE ROLE OF DIET IN MAST CELL ACTIVATION SYNDROME (MCAS)

The role of diet in Mast Cell Activation Syndrome (MCAS) is a critical component of managing this complex condition. The relationship between diet and MCAS revolves around identifying and minimizing triggers that activate mast cells, subsequently causing the release of inflammatory mediators.

Histamine-Restricted Diet:

Avoidance of High-Histamine Foods: Histamine is a crucial mediator in mast cell activation, and some individuals with MCAS find relief by limiting their intake of high-histamine foods. These may include fermented foods (such as sauerkraut and kimchi), aged cheeses, processed meats, and certain fruits and vegetables.

Fresh and Low-Histamine Alternatives: Choosing fresh foods and low-histamine alternatives can be beneficial. Freshly prepared meals reduce the intake of histamine and other biogenic amines.

Individualized Triggers:

Keeping a Food Diary: Maintaining a detailed food diary can help individuals with MCAS identify specific dietary triggers unique to their condition. This involves tracking food intake and correlating it with symptom occurrence.

Working with a Dietitian: Collaborating with a registered dietitian experienced in MCAS can be invaluable. A dietitian can provide guidance on creating an individualized diet plan tailored to the person's specific sensitivities and nutritional needs.

Anti-Inflammatory Diet:

Emphasis on Whole Foods: An anti-inflammatory diet rich in fruits, vegetables, whole grains, and healthy fats may help mitigate overall inflammation in the body. This can be particularly beneficial for individuals with MCAS, as chronic inflammation may contribute to mast cell activation.

Avoidance of Trigger Foods:

Identifying Specific Triggers: In addition to histamine, other compounds in foods, such as salicylates, amines, and certain additives, may trigger mast cell activation in some individuals. Identifying and avoiding these specific triggers can be crucial for symptom management.

Hydration and Nutritional Support:

Adequate Hydration: Staying well-hydrated is essential for individuals with MCAS. Proper hydration can support overall health and help flush out histamine and other mediators from the body.

Nutritional Supplements: In some cases, dietary supplements may be recommended to address specific nutritional deficiencies or support overall health. However, supplementation should be approached with caution and under the guidance of a healthcare professional.

CHALLENGES AND CONSIDERATIONS

Several key challenges and considerations include:

Difficulty in Maintaining a Restrictive Diet:

Social and Practical Challenges: Adopting and adhering to a restrictive diet, such as a low-histamine or anti-inflammatory diet, can be challenging in social settings or when dining out. Individuals with MCAS may face difficulties finding suitable food options that align with their dietary restrictions.

Emotional Impact: The emotional impact of restrictive diets should not be underestimated. Feelings of frustration, isolation, and anxiety related to food choices can arise, impacting the overall well-being of individuals with MCAS.

Balancing Nutritional Needs While Avoiding Triggers:

Potential Nutrient Deficiencies: Dietary restrictions aimed at avoiding triggers, particularly in a histamine-restricted diet, may pose challenges in obtaining a balanced and diverse array of nutrients. Nutrient deficiencies can impact overall health, and careful consideration is needed to address nutritional needs.

Consultation with Dietitians: Collaboration with registered dietitians experienced in MCAS management is essential. These professionals can provide guidance on creating a well-rounded diet that meets nutritional requirements while avoiding trigger foods.

Importance of Regular Follow-up with Healthcare Providers:

Dynamic Nature of MCAS: MCAS is an emotional condition, and individual responses to triggers, symptoms, and treatment strategies can change over time. Regular follow-up appointments with healthcare providers, including allergists, immunologists, and other specialists, are crucial to assess the effectiveness of the current management plan and make necessary adjustments.

Monitoring Medications and Side Effects: Medications prescribed to manage MCAS symptoms may require regular monitoring for efficacy and potential side effects. Close communication with healthcare providers allows for timely adjustments and optimization of medication regimens.

Addressing Emerging Challenges: As new challenges arise, whether related to symptom patterns, lifestyle adjustments, or emotional well-being, regular follow-ups provide a platform for individuals to discuss concerns and work collaboratively with their healthcare team to address evolving needs.

Psychosocial Considerations:

Impact on Mental Health: Living with MCAS can have a significant effect on mental health. The challenges of managing symptoms, dietary restrictions, and the unpredictability of the condition can contribute to stress and anxiety. Psychosocial support, including counseling and support groups, can be valuable in addressing these aspects of the condition.

Holistic Wellness: Recognizing the interconnectedness of physical and mental health is crucial. Integrating strategies for stress management, emotional well-being, and a holistic approach to wellness is an essential consideration in the overall management of MCAS.

CHAPTER TWO

Low Histamine Diet Recipes

Grilled Lemon-Herbed Chicken Breast

Meal Description:

This Grilled Lemon-Herbed Chicken Breast recipe offers a burst of fresh flavors with zesty lemon and aromatic herbs. It's a simple yet delicious meal that's perfect for a quick and healthy dinner.

Ingredients:

- Four boneless, skinless chicken breasts
- Two tablespoons of olive oil
- Zest of 1 lemon
- Juice of 2 lemons
- Two cloves garlic, minced
- One teaspoon dried oregano
- One teaspoon of dried thyme
- One teaspoon of dried rosemary
- Salt and pepper, to taste
- Lemon slices (for garnish)

Instructions:

Prepare the Marinade:

In a small bowl, combine olive oil, lemon zest, lemon juice, minced garlic, oregano, thyme, rosemary, salt, and pepper. Mix well to create a marinade.

Marinate the Chicken:

Place the chicken breasts in a resealable plastic bag

or shallow dish.

Pour half of the marinade over the chicken, ensuring each piece is well-coated.

Seal the bag or cover the dish and refrigerate for at least 30 minutes (or up to 4 hours for more flavor).

Preheat the Grill:

Preheat the grill to medium-high heat.

Grill the Chicken:

Remove the chicken from the marinade, letting excess drip off.

Place the chicken on the preheated grill and cook for 6-8 minutes per side or until the internal temperature reaches 165°F (74°C) and the chicken is no longer pink in the center.

Baste with Reserved Marinade:

While grilling, baste the chicken with the reserved marinade for added flavor.

Serve:

Once cooked through, remove the chicken from the grill and let it rest for a few minutes.

Garnish with lemon slices and serve.

Nutrition Information (per serving):

- Calories: 220

- Protein: 30g

- Carbohydrates: 3g

- Fat: 9g

- Saturated Fat: 1.5g

- Cholesterol: 80mg
- Sodium: 350mg
- Fiber: 1g
- Sugar: 0g

BAKED SALMON WITH DILL AND OLIVE OIL

Meal Description:

This Baked Salmon with Dill and Olive Oil is a delightful and heart-healthy dish that combines the rich flavor of salmon with the freshness of dill and the richness of olive oil. This recipe is delicious and a quick and easy way to incorporate omega-3 fatty acids into your diet.

Ingredients:

- Four salmon fillets
- Two tablespoons of olive oil
- Two tablespoons fresh dill, chopped
- Two cloves garlic, minced
- One lemon, thinly sliced
- Salt and pepper, to taste
- Lemon wedges (for serving)

Instructions:

Preheat the Oven:

Preheat your oven to 375°F (190°C).

Prepare the Salmon:

Pat the salmon fillets dry with a paper towel and place them on a baking sheet lined with parchment paper.

Season the Salmon:

Drizzle the olive oil over the salmon fillets, ensuring they are well-coated.

Sprinkle chopped dill and minced garlic evenly over the fillets.

Season with salt and pepper to taste.

Add Lemon Slices:

Place lemon slices on top of each salmon fillet for a burst of citrus flavor.

Bake in the Oven:

Bake in the preheated oven for 12-15 minutes or until the salmon is cooked through and flakes easily with a fork.

Broil for Crispy Top (Optional):

For a slightly crispy top, switch the oven to broil for the last 2-3 minutes of cooking. Keep a close eye to prevent burning.

Serve:

Carefully transfer the baked salmon to plates.

Garnish with additional fresh dill and serve with lemon wedges on the side.

Nutrition Information (per serving):

• Calories: 280

- Protein: 34g
- Carbohydrates: 2g
- Fat: 15g
- Saturated Fat: 2.5g
- Cholesterol: 90mg
- Sodium: 75mg
- Fiber: 1g
- Sugar: 0g

QUINOA SALAD WITH FRESH CUCUMBER AND AVOCADO

Meal Description:

This Quinoa Salad with Fresh Cucumber and Avocado is a vibrant and nutritious dish that combines the wholesome goodness of quinoa with the crispiness of cucumber and the creamy texture of avocado. Packed with fresh ingredients and tossed in a zesty dressing, this salad perfectly balances flavors and textures.

Ingredients:

- 1 cup quinoa, cooked and cooled

- One cucumber, diced

- 1 ripe avocado, diced

- 1 cup cherry tomatoes, halved

- 1/4 cup red onion, finely chopped

- 1/4 cup fresh cilantro, chopped

- Juice of 1 lemon

- Two tablespoons of olive oil

- One clove garlic, minced

- Salt and pepper, to taste

Instructions:

Prepare the Quinoa:

Cook quinoa according to package instructions. Once cooked, let it cool to room temperature.

Chop Fresh Ingredients:

Dice the cucumber and avocado into bite-sized pieces.

Halve the cherry tomatoes.

Finely chop the red onion and fresh cilantro.

Combine Ingredients:

Combine the cooked quinoa, diced cucumber, avocado, cherry tomatoes, red onion, and chopped cilantro in a large bowl.

Prepare the Dressing:

Whisk together lemon juice, olive oil, minced garlic, salt, and pepper in a small bowl.

Toss Salad:

Pour the dressing over the quinoa mixture.

Gently toss the salad until all ingredients are well coated with the dressing.

Chill and Serve:

For optimal flavor, refrigerate the quinoa salad for at least 30 minutes before serving.

Serve chilled, garnished with additional cilantro if desired.

Nutrition Information (per serving):

- Calories: 320

- Protein: 7g

- Carbohydrates: 35g

- Fat: 18g

- Saturated Fat: 2.5g

- Cholesterol: 0mg

- Sodium: 15mg

- Fiber: 7g

- Sugar: 2g

STIR-FRIED BOK CHOY WITH GINGER AND GARLIC

Meal Description:

This Stir-Fried Bok Choy with Ginger and Garlic is a quick and flavorful side dish that highlights the crisp texture of bok choy along with the aromatic blend of ginger and garlic. It's a delightful accompaniment to any Asian-inspired meal and adds a burst of freshness to your plate.

Ingredients:

• Four baby bok choy heads, cleaned and halved

• Two tablespoons of vegetable oil

• Two teaspoons fresh ginger, minced

• Two cloves garlic, minced

• One tablespoon of soy sauce

• One teaspoon sesame oil

• One teaspoon of rice vinegar

• 1/2 teaspoon sugar (optional)

• Red pepper flakes (optional, for heat)

• Sesame seeds, for garnish

• Green onions, sliced, for garnish

Instructions:

Prepare Bok Choy:

Trim the ends of the bok choy and cut each head in half lengthwise. Rinse under cold water to remove any dirt.

Heat the Wok or Pan:

Heat vegetable oil in a wok or large pan over medium-high heat.

Add Ginger and Garlic:

Add minced ginger and garlic to the hot oil. Stir-fry for about 30 seconds until fragrant but not browned.

Stir-Fry Bok Choy:

Add the bok choy halves to the wok cut side down. Cook for 2-3 minutes until the edges begin to brown.

Prepare Sauce:

In a small bowl, mix soy sauce, sesame oil, rice vinegar, and sugar (if using). Adjust the sauce to your taste.

Add Sauce to Wok:

Pour the sauce over the bok choy. Toss to coat evenly, ensuring the bok choy is well-cooked but still crisp.

Optional Heat:

Add red pepper flakes if you desire a bit of heat. Toss to incorporate.

Garnish and Serve:

Transfer the stir-fried bok choy to a serving platter.

Garnish with sesame seeds and sliced green onions.

Nutrition Information (per serving):

- Calories: 80

- Protein: 2g

- Carbohydrates: 7g

- Fat: 6g

- Saturated Fat: 0.5g

- Cholesterol: 0mg

- Sodium: 380mg

- Fiber: 2g

- Sugar: 2g

ZUCCHINI NOODLES WITH PESTO SAUCE

Meal Description:

Zucchini Noodles with Pesto Sauce is a light, low-carb alternative to traditional pasta dishes. This quick and easy recipe combines spiralized zucchini with a vibrant and flavorful homemade pesto sauce for a delicious and nutritious meal.

Ingredients:

For Zucchini Noodles:

• Four medium-sized zucchinis, spiralized

• One tablespoon of olive oil

• Salt and pepper, to taste

For Pesto Sauce:

• 2 cups fresh basil leaves, packed

• 1/2 cup grated Parmesan cheese

• 1/2 cup pine nuts or walnuts

• Three cloves garlic peeled

• 1/2 cup extra-virgin olive oil

• Salt and pepper, to taste

• Juice of 1 lemon (optional)

Instructions:

Prepare Zucchini Noodles:

Spiralize the zucchinis to create noodle-like strands. If you don't have a spiralizer, you can use a vegetable peeler to make thin ribbons.

Heat olive oil in a large pan over medium heat. Add zucchini noodles, season with salt and pepper, and sauté for 2-3 minutes until just tender. Be careful not to overcook; you want the noodles to maintain a slight crunch.

Make Pesto Sauce:

Combine basil, grated Parmesan, pine nuts or walnuts, and garlic in a food processor. Pulse until coarsely chopped.

With the food processor running, slowly pour in the olive oil until the pesto reaches a smooth consistency. Season with salt and pepper to taste. Add lemon juice if desired for a citrusy kick.

Combine Zucchini Noodles and Pesto:

Toss the sautéed zucchini noodles with the freshly made pesto sauce until well-coated.

Serve:

Divide the zucchini noodles into serving plates.

Optionally, garnish with additional grated Parmesan and a sprinkle of pine nuts.

Serve immediately, and enjoy the light and

refreshing flavors.

Nutrition Information (per serving):

• Calories: 280

• Protein: 7g

• Carbohydrates: 10g

• Fat: 25g

• Saturated Fat: 4g

• Cholesterol: 5mg

• Sodium: 200mg

• Fiber: 4g

• Sugar: 5g

FRESH MANGO SALSA

Meal Description:

This Fresh Mango Salsa is a burst of tropical flavors that add a refreshing and vibrant touch to various dishes. Whether paired with grilled chicken or fish tacos or enjoyed with tortilla chips, this easy-to-make salsa is a delightful combination of sweet and savory.

Ingredients:

- Two ripe mangoes, peeled, pitted, and diced
- One red bell pepper, finely diced
- 1/2 red onion, finely chopped
- One jalapeño, seeded and finely minced
- 1/4 cup fresh cilantro, chopped
- Juice of 2 limes
- Salt and pepper, to taste

Instructions:

Prepare the Mangoes:

Peel, pit, and dice the ripe mangoes. If you need to become more familiar with cutting mangoes, you can find tutorials online to help you navigate around the pit.

Dice Vegetables:

Finely dice the red bell pepper and red onion.

Seed and finely mince the jalapeño. Adjust the amount based on your desired level of heat.

Chop Cilantro:

Chop fresh cilantro leaves. If you're not a fan of cilantro, you can substitute it with fresh parsley.

Combine Ingredients:

Combine the diced mangoes, red bell pepper, red onion, minced jalapeño, and chopped cilantro in a bowl.

Add Lime Juice:

Squeeze the juice of two limes over the mixture. Adjust the amount to your taste preference.

Season with Salt and Pepper:

Season the salsa with salt and pepper. Be mindful of the saltiness, as you can always add more later.

Mix Well:

Gently toss all the ingredients until well combined. Ensure the lime juice evenly coats the mixture.

Chill (Optional):

Let the salsa chill in the refrigerator for about 30 minutes before serving for enhanced flavors.

Serve:

Serve the Fresh Mango Salsa as a topping for grilled proteins, fish tacos, or as a refreshing dip with tortilla chips.

Serving Suggestion:

• Pair with grilled chicken, fish, or shrimp.

• Spoon over tacos or quesadillas.

• Enjoy as a standalone salsa with tortilla chips.

Nutrition Information (per serving):

• Calories: 60

• Protein: 1g

• Carbohydrates: 15g

• Fat: 0.5g

• Saturated Fat: 0g

• Cholesterol: 0mg

• Sodium: 5mg

• Fiber: 2g

• Sugar: 11g

ROASTED TURKEY BREAST WITH ROSEMARY

Meal Description:

This Roasted Turkey Breast with Rosemary is a classic and elegant dish that brings out the rich flavors of turkey enhanced by the earthy aroma of fresh rosemary. Whether you're preparing a holiday feast or a special dinner, this recipe ensures a moist and flavorful turkey breast with minimal fuss.

Ingredients:

• One whole bone-in turkey breast (about 5-6 pounds)

• Three tablespoons olive oil

• Three cloves garlic, minced

• One tablespoon of fresh rosemary, finely chopped

• One teaspoon of dried thyme

• One teaspoon paprika

• Salt and black pepper, to taste

• 1 cup chicken or turkey broth

Instructions:

Preheat the Oven:

Preheat your oven to 325°F (163°C).

Prepare the Turkey Breast:

Rinse the turkey breast under cold water and pat it dry with paper towels. Place it on a roasting rack set inside a roasting pan.

Season the Turkey:

Mix olive oil, minced garlic, chopped rosemary, thyme, paprika, salt, and black pepper in a small bowl to create a paste.

Rub the turkey breast with the seasoning paste, ensuring it's evenly coated.

Tie the turkey:

If your turkey breast comes untied, use kitchen twine to secure it in a neat, compact shape. This promotes even cooking.

Roast Turkey:

Place the roasting pan in the preheated oven. Roast the turkey breast, basting with pan juices every 30 minutes, until the internal temperature reaches 165°F (74°C). This typically takes about 2 to 2.5 hours, depending on the size of the turkey.

Add Broth:

About halfway through the cooking time, add the chicken or turkey broth to the bottom of the roasting pan. This helps keep the turkey moist and enhances the flavor.

Check for Doneness:

Use a meat thermometer to check the turkey's internal temperature in the thickest part of the breast. Once it reaches 165°F (74°C), the turkey is done.

Rest the Turkey:

Remove the turkey from the oven and let it rest for 15-20 minutes before carving. This redistributes the juices, ensuring a moist and flavorful turkey.

Carve and Serve:

Carve the turkey breast into slices and arrange on a serving platter. Garnish with additional fresh rosemary if desired.

Serving Suggestions:

• Serve with your favorite gravy.

• Pair with cranberry sauce for a classic combination.

• Accompany with roasted vegetables or mashed potatoes.

Nutrition Information (per serving):

• Calories: 250

• Protein: 35g

• Carbohydrates: 0g

• Fat: 12g

• Saturated Fat: 2.5g

• Cholesterol: 95mg

• Sodium: 300mg

• Fiber: 0g

• Sugar: 0g

STEAMED ASPARAGUS WITH LEMON ZEST

Meal Description:

This Steamed Asparagus with Lemon Zest is a simple yet elegant side dish that highlights the fresh and vibrant flavors of asparagus. Steaming preserves the natural crispness of the asparagus, and the addition of lemon zest provides a zesty and refreshing twist.

Ingredients:

- One bunch of fresh asparagus, tough ends trimmed
- One tablespoon of olive oil
- Zest of 1 lemon
- Salt and pepper, to taste
- Lemon wedges for serving (optional)

Instructions:

Prepare the Asparagus:

Wash the asparagus under cold water. Trim the tough ends by snapping or cutting them off.

Steam the Asparagus:

In a steamer basket over boiling water, steam the asparagus for 3-5 minutes or until it becomes bright green and tender but still crisp. Cooking time may vary depending on the thickness of the asparagus spears.

Prepare Lemon Zest:

While the asparagus is steaming, use a zester or fine grater to zest the lemon. Be careful to zest the yellow part, avoiding the bitter white pith.

Toss with Olive Oil:

Once the asparagus is steamed, transfer it to a serving platter. Drizzle with olive oil and toss gently to coat.

Add Lemon Zest:

Sprinkle the lemon zest evenly over the steamed asparagus. The lemon zest adds a burst of citrus flavor and aroma.

Season with Salt and Pepper:

Season the asparagus with salt and pepper to taste. Toss once more to ensure even seasoning.

Serve:

Arrange the steamed asparagus on a serving plate. Optionally, serve with lemon wedges on the side for an extra citrusy kick.

Serving Suggestions:

Serve as a side dish for grilled chicken or fish.

Pair with a poached egg for a light and nutritious breakfast.

Include in a vegetable medley as part of a colorful dinner spread.

Nutrition Information (per serving):

- Calories: 40

- Protein: 2g

- Carbohydrates: 4g

- Fat: 3g

- Saturated Fat: 0.5g

- Cholesterol: 0mg

- Sodium: 0mg

- Fiber: 2g

- Sugar: 2g

TURKEY AND VEGETABLE SKEWERS

Meal Description:

These Turkey and Vegetable Skewers are a delicious and colorful way to enjoy a balanced, protein-packed meal. Grilled to perfection, these skewers feature tender turkey chunks paired with a medley of vibrant vegetables, creating a flavorful and visually appealing dish.

Ingredients:

• 1 pound turkey breast, cut into bite-sized chunks

• One zucchini, sliced into rounds

• One red bell pepper, cut into chunks

• One yellow bell pepper, cut into chunks

• One red onion, cut into wedges

• Cherry tomatoes

• Two tablespoons of olive oil

• Two cloves garlic, minced

• One teaspoon dried oregano

• One teaspoon of dried thyme

- Salt and pepper, to taste
- Wooden skewers, soaked in water for 30 minutes

Instructions:

Prepare the Marinade:

Mix olive oil, minced garlic, dried oregano, dried thyme, salt, and pepper to create a marinade in a bowl.

Marinate the turkey:

Place the turkey chunks in the marinade, ensuring they are well-coated. Allow to marinate for at least 30 minutes to let the flavors infuse.

Assemble the Skewers:

Preheat the grill to medium-high heat.

Thread the marinated turkey chunks, zucchini rounds, bell pepper chunks, red onion wedges, and cherry tomatoes onto the soaked wooden skewers, alternating between turkey and vegetables.

Grill the Skewers:

Place the assembled skewers on the preheated grill. Cook for 10-12 minutes, turning occasionally, until the turkey is cooked and the vegetables are charred and tender.

Serve:

Remove the skewers from the grill and transfer them to a serving platter.

Optionally, garnish with fresh herbs, such as chopped parsley or cilantro.

Serving Suggestions:

Serve over a bed of cooked quinoa or rice.

Drizzle with a light lemon vinaigrette or tzatziki sauce.

Pair with a side salad for a complete and well-balanced meal.

Nutrition Information (per serving):

• Calories: 220

• Protein: 25g

• Carbohydrates: 10g

• Fat: 9g

• Saturated Fat: 1.5g

• Cholesterol: 50mg

• Sodium: 70mg

• Fiber: 3g

• Sugar: 5g

COCONUT MILK SMOOTHIE WITH FRESH BERRIES

Smoothie Description:

This Coconut Milk Smoothie with Fresh Berries is a tropical delight that combines the rich creaminess of coconut milk with the vibrant flavors of fresh berries. Packed with antioxidants, this smoothie is delicious and a nutritious and refreshing treat.

Ingredients:

• 1 cup coconut milk (canned, unsweetened)

• 1 cup mixed fresh berries (strawberries, blueberries, raspberries)

• One ripe banana, peeled and sliced

• One tablespoon of chia seeds (optional for added texture)

• One tablespoon of honey or maple syrup (optional for sweetness)

• Ice cubes (optional)

• Shredded coconut for garnish (optional)

Instructions:

Prepare Ingredients:

Wash the fresh berries and slice the banana.

Blend the Smoothie:

In a blender, combine coconut milk, mixed berries, sliced banana, chia seeds (if using), and honey or maple syrup (if desired).

You can add a handful of ice cubes if you prefer a colder smoothie.

Blend Until Smooth:

Blend the ingredients until smooth and creamy. If the consistency is too thick, you can add more coconut milk to achieve your preferred thickness.

Taste and Adjust:

Taste the smoothie and adjust the sweetness if needed by adding more honey or maple syrup.

Serve:

Pour the smoothie into glasses and garnish with shredded coconut if desired.

Enjoy:

Sip and savor the tropical flavors of this Coconut Milk Smoothie with Fresh Berries.

Serving Suggestions:

Top with additional fresh berries for an extra burst of flavor.

Sprinkle with granola or nuts for added crunch.

• Enjoy as a refreshing breakfast or snack.

Nutrition Information (per serving):

- Calories: 250
- Protein: 3g
- Carbohydrates: 30g
- Fat: 14g
- Saturated Fat: 11g
- Cholesterol: 0mg
- Sodium: 20mg
- Fiber: 6g
- Sugar: 18g

RICE CAKE WITH AVOCADO AND SEA SALT

Snack Description:

This Rice Cake with Avocado and Sea Salt is a quick, wholesome, and satisfying snack that combines the creamy texture of ripe avocado with the crunch of a rice cake. Topped with a sprinkle of sea salt, it's a delightful balance of flavors and textures.

Ingredients:

• One rice cake (whole grain or your preferred variety)

• 1/2 ripe avocado, sliced

• Sea salt, to taste

• Optional toppings: red pepper flakes, lemon juice, or a drizzle of balsamic glaze

Instructions:

Prepare Avocado:

Slice the ripe avocado and scoop out the flesh.

Assemble the Snack:

Place a rice cake on a plate or a flat surface.

Layer with Avocado:

Arrange the avocado slices on top of the rice cake, ensuring even coverage.

Season with Sea Salt:

Sprinkle sea salt over the avocado to enhance the flavor. Be mindful not to oversalt; you can always add more later.

Optional Toppings:

If desired, add additional toppings like a pinch of red pepper flakes for a hint of heat, a squeeze of fresh lemon juice for acidity, or a drizzle of balsamic glaze for added sweetness.

Serve Immediately:

Enjoy your Rice Cake with Avocado and Sea Salt immediately for the best combination of textures.

Serving Suggestions:

Pair with a cup of herbal tea for a light and satisfying snack.

Customize with additional toppings like cherry tomatoes, radishes, or microgreens for added freshness.

Serve as part of a balanced breakfast or as a quick midday pick-me-up.

Nutrition Information (per serving):

- Calories: 150

- Protein: 2g

- Carbohydrates: 12g

- Fat: 11g

- Saturated Fat: 1.5g
- Cholesterol: 0mg
- Sodium: 150mg
- Fiber: 5g
- Sugar: 0.5g

FRESH STRAWBERRIES WITH COCONUT CREAM

Dessert Description:

Fresh Strawberries with Coconut Cream is a simple yet indulgent dessert that celebrates the natural sweetness of ripe strawberries paired with the velvety richness of coconut cream. This delightful treat is a refreshing and dairy-free option for those seeking a luscious and guilt-free dessert.

Ingredients:

• 1 cup fresh strawberries, hulled and halved

• 1/2 cup coconut cream (chilled)

• One tablespoon of maple syrup or agave nectar

• Shredded coconut for garnish (optional)

• Fresh mint leaves for garnish (optional)

Instructions:

Prepare Strawberries:

Wash, hull, and halve the fresh strawberries. You

can leave a few strawberries whole for garnish for an elegant presentation.

Chill Coconut Cream:

Place the can of coconut cream in the refrigerator for at least 4 hours or overnight. This helps separate the cream from the liquid.

Extract Coconut Cream:

Open the chilled can of coconut cream without shaking. Scoop out the thickened cream from the top of the can, leaving the liquid behind.

Whip Coconut Cream:

In a mixing bowl, whip the coconut cream using a hand mixer or whisk until it reaches a smooth and fluffy consistency.

Sweeten Coconut Cream:

Add maple syrup or agave nectar to the whipped coconut cream. Adjust the sweetness to your liking and mix until well combined.

Assemble Dessert:

Place the halved strawberries in serving bowls or plates.

Top with Coconut Cream:

Spoon the sweetened coconut cream generously over the fresh strawberries.

Garnish:

Garnish with shredded coconut for added texture and freshness. Optionally, add a few whole strawberries and mint leaves for a decorative touch.

Serve Immediately:

Serve Fresh Strawberries with Coconut Cream immediately for the best taste and texture.

Serving Suggestions:

Pair with a sprinkle of crushed nuts, such as almonds or pistachios, for added crunch.

Enjoy as a light and satisfying dessert after a meal.

Serve alongside a scoop of dairy-free vanilla ice cream for an extra treat.

Nutrition Information (per serving):

- Calories: 180

- Protein: 1g

- Carbohydrates: 12g

- Fat: 15g

- Saturated Fat: 13g

- Cholesterol: 0mg

- Sodium: 10mg

- Fiber: 3g

- Sugar: 7g

RICE PAPER ROLLS WITH SHRIMP AND FRESH VEGETABLES

Appetizer/Snack Description:

Rice Paper Rolls with Shrimp and Fresh Vegetables are light, refreshing, and full of vibrant flavors. These translucent rolls are filled with succulent shrimp, crisp vegetables, and vermicelli noodles, creating a delicious appetizer or snack. Served with a flavorful dipping sauce, they make a perfect addition to any gathering.

Ingredients:

For Rice Paper Rolls:

- Eight rice paper sheets (spring roll wrappers)
- 16 medium-sized cooked shrimp, peeled and deveined
- 1 cup vermicelli noodles, cooked and cooled
- 1 cup lettuce leaves, shredded
- 1 cup cucumber, julienned
- One carrot, julienned
- Fresh mint leaves
- Fresh cilantro leaves

For Dipping Sauce:

- 1/4 cup hoisin sauce

- Two tablespoons of soy sauce

- One tablespoon of rice vinegar

- One teaspoon sesame oil

- One teaspoon honey

- Crushed peanuts for garnish (optional)

Instructions:

Prepare Ingredients:

Cook and peel the shrimp. Cook the vermicelli noodles according to package instructions, then cool them under running water. Julienne the cucumber and carrot. Shred the lettuce.

Create a Dipping Station:

Fill a large shallow bowl with warm water. Place all prepared ingredients within easy reach on a clean work surface.

Soak Rice Paper Sheets:

Dip one rice paper sheet into the warm water, ensuring it is fully submerged. Rotate for about 10-15 seconds until it softens.

Assemble the Rice Paper Rolls:

Place the softened rice paper sheet on a flat surface.

In the center, add a few shrimp, a handful of vermicelli noodles, shredded lettuce, julienned cucumber and carrot, mint leaves, and cilantro leaves.

Roll the Rice Paper:

Fold the sides of the rice paper over the filling, then fold the bottom over the filling and tightly roll it up from the bottom to the top.

Repeat:

Repeat the process with the remaining rice paper sheets and filling ingredients.

Prepare Dipping Sauce:

Mix hoisin sauce, soy sauce, rice vinegar, sesame oil, and honey in a small bowl. Adjust the ingredients to taste.

Serve:

Arrange the Rice Paper Rolls on a serving platter, and sprinkle crushed peanuts on top optionally.

Serve with the prepared dipping sauce.

Serving Suggestions:

These rolls can be served as appetizers, snacks, or light meals.

Pair with a side of sweet chili sauce for an extra kick.

Customize the filling with your favorite herbs, such as basil or Thai basil.

Nutrition Information (per serving - 2 rolls with dipping sauce):

• Calories: 250

• Protein: 15g

• Carbohydrates: 40g

- Fat: 3g
- Saturated Fat: 0.5g
- Cholesterol: 80mg
- Sodium: 600mg
- Fiber: 3g
- Sugar: 6g

BAKED SWEET POTATO CHIPS

Snack Description:

These Baked Sweet Potato Chips are a healthier alternative to traditional potato chips, offering a crispy texture and sweet flavor. Simple to make, these chips are seasoned with a hint of salt and can be enjoyed as a guilt-free snack or a crunchy side dish.

Ingredients:

- Two large sweet potatoes peeled

- Two tablespoons of olive oil

- One teaspoon salt

- 1/2 teaspoon paprika (optional for added flavor)

- 1/2 teaspoon garlic powder (optional for added flavor)

- Freshly ground black pepper, to taste

Instructions:

Preheat the Oven:

Preheat your oven to 375°F (190°C).

Slice the Sweet Potatoes:

Thinly slice the peeled sweet potatoes using a sharp knife or a mandoline slicer. Aim for uniform thickness to ensure even baking.

Soak in Cold Water:

Soak the sweet potato slices in a bowl of cold water for about 30 minutes. This helps remove excess starch and contributes to crispiness.

Dry Thoroughly:

Drain the sweet potato slices and pat them completely dry with paper towels.

Season the Chips:

In a large bowl, toss the sweet potato slices with olive oil, salt, and any optional seasonings such as paprika and garlic powder. Ensure each slice is evenly coated.

Arrange on Baking Sheets:

Place a wire rack on each baking sheet to allow air circulation. Arrange the seasoned sweet potato slices in a single layer on the wire racks.

Bake:

Bake in the preheated oven for 15-20 minutes or until the edges of the chips are golden brown and crisp. Be vigilant to prevent burning.

Cool and Serve:

Allow the sweet potato chips to cool on the wire racks. They will continue to crisp up as they cool.

Season to Taste:

Once cooled, taste a chip and add additional salt or pepper if needed.

Serve:

Serve the Baked Sweet Potato Chips as a snack, appetizer, or a healthier alternative to traditional potato chips.

Serving Suggestions:

Pair with a yogurt-based dip or guacamole for added flavor.

Enjoy alongside a sandwich or wrap for a crunchy side.

Sprinkle with a pinch of smoked paprika for a smoky twist.

Nutrition Information (per serving):

• Calories: 120

• Protein: 1g

• Carbohydrates: 18g

• Fat: 5g

• Saturated Fat: 0.5g

• Cholesterol: 0mg

• Sodium: 480mg

• Fiber: 3g

• Sugar: 5g

ALMOND BUTTER AND BANANA SMOOTHIE BOWL

Bowl Description:

This Almond Butter and Banana Smoothie Bowl is a creamy, satisfying breakfast or snack option. Packed with wholesome ingredients, it combines the richness of almond butter with the natural sweetness of bananas. Topped with a variety of nutritious add-ins, it's a delicious and nourishing way to start your day.

Ingredients:

For the Smoothie Bowl:

• Two ripe bananas frozen

• Two tablespoons of almond butter

• 1/2 cup unsweetened almond milk (or your preferred milk)

• One tablespoon of chia seeds

• One teaspoon of honey or maple syrup (optional for added sweetness)

• Ice cubes (optional for a thicker consistency)

Toppings:

- Sliced banana

- Granola

- Chopped almonds

- Shredded coconut

- Drizzle of almond butter

- Fresh berries (optional)

Instructions:

Prepare the Smoothie Base:

In a blender, combine the frozen bananas, almond butter, almond milk, chia seeds, and honey or maple syrup (if using). Blend until smooth and creamy. Add ice cubes if you prefer a thicker consistency.

Pour into a Bowl:

Pour the smoothie into a bowl, ensuring it has a thick and spoonable texture.

Add Toppings:

Decorate the smoothie bowl with sliced banana, granola, chopped almonds, shredded coconut, and any other toppings of your choice.

Drizzle with Almond Butter:

Finish the bowl with a generous drizzle of almond butter for added richness and flavor.

Customize:

Get creative with your toppings; add fresh berries, seeds, or a sprinkle of cinnamon for extra flair.

Serve Immediately:

Enjoy your Almond Butter and Banana Smoothie Bowl immediately, savoring the combination of creamy smoothie and crunchy toppings.

Serving Suggestions:

Customize with your favorite fruits, nuts, or seeds.

Top with a dollop of Greek yogurt for added protein.

Enjoy as a post-workout snack or a satisfying breakfast.

Nutrition Information (approximate values):

- Calories: 450

- Protein: 10g

- Carbohydrates: 50g

- Fat: 25g

- Saturated Fat: 2g

- Cholesterol: 0mg

- Sodium: 80mg

- Fiber: 10g

- Sugar: 24g

CHAPTER THREE

Anti-Inflammatory Diet Recipes

Turmeric-Ginger Carrot Soup

Soup Description:

This turmeric ginger Carrot Soup is a comforting and nourishing dish that brings together the earthy sweetness of carrots with the warmth of turmeric and ginger. Packed with antioxidants and anti-inflammatory ingredients, this soup is delicious and a health-boosting option for any meal.

Ingredients:

- 1 pound carrots, peeled and sliced

- One onion, diced

- Three cloves garlic, minced

- One tablespoon of fresh ginger, grated

- One teaspoon of ground turmeric

- 1/2 teaspoon ground cumin

- 1/4 teaspoon ground coriander

- 4 cups vegetable broth

- One can (14 ounces) coconut milk

- Two tablespoons of olive oil

- Salt and pepper, to taste

- Fresh cilantro or parsley for garnish (optional)

Instructions:

Prepare the Vegetables:

Peel and slice the carrots. Dice the onion, mince the garlic, and grate the fresh ginger.

Sauté Aromatics:

In a large pot, heat olive oil over medium heat. Add the diced onion and cook until softened about 5 minutes.

Add Garlic and Ginger:

Stir in the minced garlic and grated ginger, cooking for an additional 1-2 minutes until fragrant.

Season with Spices:

Sprinkle ground turmeric, ground cumin, and ground coriander over the aromatics. Stir to coat the vegetables in the spices.

Add Carrots:

Add the sliced carrots to the pot, stirring to combine with the aromatic and spice mixture.

Pour in Vegetable Broth:

Pour in the vegetable broth, ensuring that the carrots are fully submerged. Bring the mixture to a boil, then reduce the heat and let it simmer until the carrots are tender about 15-20 minutes.

Blend the Soup:

Use an immersion blender to blend the soup until smooth. Alternatively, transfer the soup in batches to a blender and blend until smooth. Exercise caution when blending hot liquids.

Incorporate Coconut Milk:

Pour in the coconut milk and stir until well combined. Simmer the soup for an additional 5 minutes to allow the flavors to meld.

Season to Taste:

Season the soup with salt and pepper, adjusting to your taste preference.

Serve:

Ladle the turmeric ginger Carrot Soup into bowls. Garnish with fresh cilantro or parsley if desired.

Serving Suggestions:

Serve with a slice of crusty bread or a side of naan.

Top with a dollop of Greek yogurt or a swirl of coconut cream for added creaminess.

Enjoy it as a starter, or pair it with a light and wholesome salad.

Nutrition Information (per serving):

- Calories: 220

- Protein: 3g

- Carbohydrates: 20g

- Fat: 15g

- Saturated Fat: 10g

- Cholesterol: 0mg

- Sodium: 650mg

- Fiber: 4g

- Sugar: 8g

SPINACH AND BERRY SALAD WITH ALMONDS

Salad Description:

This Spinach and Berry Salad with Almonds is a delightful blend of fresh spinach, juicy berries, and crunchy almonds. Tossed in a light vinaigrette, this salad offers a perfect balance of sweet and savory flavors, making it a refreshing and nutritious choice for a light meal or a side dish.

Ingredients:

For the Salad:

- 6 cups fresh baby spinach
- 1 cup strawberries, hulled and sliced
- 1 cup blueberries
- 1/2 cup sliced almonds, toasted
- 1/4 cup crumbled feta cheese (optional)
- 1/4 cup red onion, thinly sliced

For the Vinaigrette:

- Three tablespoons extra-virgin olive oil

- Two tablespoons of balsamic vinegar

- One tablespoon honey

- One teaspoon of Dijon mustard

- Salt and pepper, to taste

Instructions:

Prepare the Salad Greens:

Wash and thoroughly dry the baby spinach. Place it in a large salad bowl.

Add Berries and Almonds:

Scatter the sliced strawberries, blueberries, and toasted sliced almonds over the bed of spinach.

Include Red Onion:

Add thinly sliced red onion to the salad for a hint of sharpness and color.

Optional Feta Cheese:

If using feta cheese, crumble it over the salad for a creamy and tangy element.

Prepare the Vinaigrette:

Whisk together extra-virgin olive oil, balsamic vinegar, honey, Dijon mustard, salt, and pepper in a small bowl. Adjust the sweetness and acidity to your taste.

Toss the Salad:

Drizzle the vinaigrette over the salad ingredients. Gently toss the salad to ensure an even coating of the vinaigrette.

Serve Immediately:

Serve the Spinach and Berry Salad with Almonds immediately, ensuring the spinach remains crisp.

Serving Suggestions:

Pair with grilled chicken or shrimp for a protein boost.

Sprinkle with chia seeds or flaxseeds for added texture and nutritional benefits.

Serve as a refreshing side dish at barbecues or picnics.

Nutrition Information (per serving):

- Calories: 200

- Protein: 4g

- Carbohydrates: 18g

- Fat: 14g

- Saturated Fat: 2g

- Cholesterol: 5mg

- Sodium: 120mg

- Fiber: 4g

- Sugar: 10g

OVEN-ROASTED BRUSSELS SPROUTS WITH TURMERIC

Side Dish Description:

These Oven-Roasted Brussels Sprouts with Turmeric are a flavorful and nutritious side dish that elevates the humble Brussels sprout to a new level. The combination of the earthy Brussels sprouts with the warm and aromatic turmeric creates a deliciously seasoned dish that is easy to prepare.

Ingredients:

- 1 pound Brussels sprouts, trimmed and halved

- 2 tablespoons olive oil

- One teaspoon of ground turmeric

- One teaspoon of garlic powder

- 1/2 teaspoon smoked paprika (optional for a smoky flavor)

- Salt and pepper, to taste

- Lemon wedges for serving

Instructions:

Preheat the Oven:

Preheat your oven to 400°F (200°C).

Prepare Brussels Sprouts:

Trim the Brussels sprouts and cut them in half, ensuring uniform sizes for even roasting.

Coat with Olive Oil:

Toss the halved Brussels sprouts with olive oil in a large bowl until they are evenly coated.

Season with Turmeric and Spices:

Sprinkle ground turmeric, garlic powder, and smoked paprika (if using) over the Brussels sprouts. Add salt and pepper to taste. Toss to coat the sprouts evenly with the spices.

Arrange on Baking Sheet:

Place the seasoned Brussels sprouts on a baking sheet in a single layer. Ensure they are open to allow for even roasting.

Roast in the Oven:

Roast in the preheated oven for 25-30 minutes or until the Brussels sprouts are golden brown and crispy on the edges. Stir halfway through the roasting time for even cooking.

Serve with Lemon Wedges:

Once roasted, transfer the Brussels sprouts to a serving dish. Serve with lemon wedges on the side for a burst of freshness.

Enjoy:

Enjoy these Oven-Roasted Brussels Sprouts with Turmeric as a flavorful and nutrient-rich side dish.

Serving Suggestions:

Pair with roasted chicken or grilled salmon for a complete meal.

Sprinkle with grated Parmesan cheese before serving for added richness.

Serve as a side dish for holiday gatherings or weeknight dinners.

Nutrition Information (per serving):

- Calories: 120
- Protein: 4g
- Carbohydrates: 12g
- Fat: 7g
- Saturated Fat: 1g
- Cholesterol: 0mg
- Sodium: 30mg
- Fiber: 5g
- Sugar: 3g

CHICKPEA AND SPINACH CURRY

Main Course Description:

Chickpea and Spinach Curry is a hearty and flavorful vegetarian dish that combines protein-rich chickpeas with spinach's vibrant goodness in a fragrant curry sauce. Packed with spices and served over rice or with naan, this curry is a wholesome and satisfying meal for any day of the week.

Ingredients:

• Two cans (15 ounces each) of chickpeas, drained and rinsed

• One onion, finely chopped

• Three cloves garlic, minced

• One tablespoon ginger, grated

• One can (14 ounces) diced tomatoes

• One large bunch of fresh spinach, washed and chopped

• One can (13.5 ounces) coconut milk

• Two tablespoons of curry powder

• One teaspoon of ground cumin

• One teaspoon of ground coriander

- 1/2 teaspoon turmeric powder
- 1/2 teaspoon red pepper flakes (adjust to taste)
- Salt and pepper, to taste
- Two tablespoons cooking oil (vegetable or coconut oil)
- Fresh cilantro, chopped, for garnish
- Cooked rice or naan for serving

Instructions:

Sauté Aromatics:

Heat the cooking oil over medium heat in a large pan or pot. Add chopped onions and sauté until they become translucent.

Add Garlic and Ginger:

Stir in minced garlic and grated ginger, cooking for an additional 1-2 minutes until fragrant.

Spice It Up:

Add curry powder, cumin, coriander, turmeric powder, and red pepper flakes to the onion mixture. Stir well to coat the aromatics in the spices.

Tomatoes and Chickpeas:

Pour in the diced tomatoes (with their juices) and add the drained and rinsed chickpeas. Stir to combine.

Simmer:

Allow the mixture to simmer for about 15-20 minutes, allowing the flavors to meld and the chickpeas to absorb the spices.

Add Coconut Milk:

Pour in the coconut milk and stir to incorporate it into the curry. Simmer for an additional 5-7 minutes.

Fold in Spinach:

Add the chopped spinach to the curry, stirring until the spinach wilts and becomes incorporated into the dish.

Season and Garnish:

Season the curry with salt and pepper according to your taste. Garnish with freshly chopped cilantro.

Serve:

Serve the Chickpea and Spinach Curry over cooked rice or with naan bread.

Serving Suggestions:

Garnish with a dollop of Greek yogurt or a squeeze of fresh lemon juice before serving.

Serve with a side of basmati rice, quinoa, or couscous for a complete meal.

Customize the spice level by adjusting the red pepper flakes or adding a sliced green chili.

Nutrition Information (per serving, without rice or naan):

- Calories: 350

- Protein: 12g

- Carbohydrates: 32g

- Fat: 20g

- Saturated Fat: 12g
- Cholesterol: 0mg
- Sodium: 600mg
- Fiber: 10g
- Sugar: 6g

GRILLED TURMERIC CHICKEN SKEWERS

Main Course Description:

Grilled Turmeric Chicken Skewers are a flavorful and aromatic dish that combines turmeric's warmth with grilled chicken's succulence. These skewers are perfect for a summer barbecue or a quick, tasty weeknight dinner. Serve with a side of rice or a fresh salad for a complete meal.

Ingredients:

For the Marinade:

• 1.5 pounds boneless, skinless chicken breasts cut into cubes

• 2 tablespoons olive oil

• One tablespoon of ground turmeric

• One teaspoon of ground cumin

• One teaspoon paprika

• One teaspoon of garlic powder

• One teaspoon of onion powder

• 1/2 teaspoon cayenne pepper (adjust to taste)

• Salt and pepper, to taste

• Juice of 1 lemon

For the Skewers:

• Wooden or metal skewers, soaked in water (if using wooden)

Instructions:

Prepare the Marinade:

In a bowl, combine olive oil, ground turmeric, ground cumin, paprika, garlic powder, onion powder, cayenne pepper, salt, pepper, and the juice of one lemon. Mix well to form a smooth marinade.

Marinate the Chicken:

Place the cubed chicken in a resealable plastic bag or shallow dish. Pour the marinade over the chicken, ensuring each piece is well coated. Marinate in the refrigerator for at least 30 minutes, or ideally, for a few hours to allow the flavors to penetrate.

Preheat the Grill:

Preheat your grill or grill pan to medium-high heat.

Skewer the Chicken:

Thread the marinated chicken cubes onto the soaked skewers, leaving a bit of space between each piece.

Grill the Skewers:

Place the skewers on the preheated grill. Grill for 12-15 minutes, turning occasionally, until the chicken is cooked through and has a nice char on the edges.

Check for Doneness:

To ensure the chicken is fully cooked, check the internal temperature using a meat thermometer. It should reach 165°F (74°C).

Serve Hot:

Remove the Grilled Turmeric Chicken Skewers from the grill and serve hot.

Serving Suggestions:

Serve with a side of mint yogurt sauce or tzatziki for dipping.

Pair with couscous, quinoa, or a fresh green salad for a well-balanced meal.

Garnish with chopped cilantro or parsley for a burst of freshness.

Nutrition Information (per serving, without sides):

• Calories: 250

• Protein: 30g

• Carbohydrates: 2g

• Fat: 14g

• Saturated Fat: 2g

• Cholesterol: 90mg

• Sodium: 350mg

• Fiber: 1g

• Sugar: 0g

SWEET POTATO AND KALE HASH

Breakfast or Brunch Dish Description:

Sweet Potato and Kale Hash is a hearty and nutritious breakfast or brunch option that combines sweet potatoes' natural sweetness with the earthy kale flavors. This one-pan dish is delicious and packed with vitamins and fiber, making it a perfect way to start your day.

Ingredients:

- Two medium sweet potatoes, peeled and diced
- One bunch of kale stems removed and leaves chopped
- One small onion, finely chopped
- 2 cloves garlic, minced
- 2 tablespoons olive oil
- One teaspoon of smoked paprika
- 1/2 teaspoon cumin
- 1/2 teaspoon paprika
- Salt and pepper, to taste
- Four eggs (optional for serving)
- Fresh parsley, chopped, for garnish

Instructions:

Prepare Sweet Potatoes:

Peel and dice the sweet potatoes into small, uniform cubes.

Sauté Onions and Garlic:

In a large skillet, heat olive oil over medium heat. Add chopped onions and minced garlic. Sauté until the onions are translucent.

Add Sweet Potatoes:

Add the diced sweet potatoes to the skillet. Cook for 10-12 minutes or until the sweet potatoes are tender, stirring occasionally.

Season with Spices:

Sprinkle smoked paprika, cumin, paprika, salt, and pepper over the sweet potatoes. Stir to coat the sweet potatoes with the spices evenly.

Incorporate Kale:

Add the chopped kale to the skillet. Cook for 5-7 minutes or until the kale is wilted and tender.

Adjust Seasoning:

Taste and adjust the seasoning if needed. Add more salt or pepper, according to your preference.

Optional: Add Eggs (Poached or Fried):

Create wells in the hash and crack eggs into them. Cover the skillet and cook until the eggs are cooked to your liking.

Garnish and Serve:

Garnish the sweet potato and kale hash with freshly chopped parsley. Serve hot, either on its own or with a side of toast.

Serving Suggestions:

Top with crumbled feta or goat cheese for added creaminess.

Serve with a dollop of Greek yogurt or a drizzle of hot sauce.

Pair with avocado slices for extra richness and flavor.

Nutrition Information (per serving, without eggs):

- Calories: 220

- Protein: 4g

- Carbohydrates: 30g

- Fat: 10g

- Saturated Fat: 1.5g

- Cholesterol: 0mg

- Sodium: 80mg

- Fiber: 5g

- Sugar: 6g

AVOCADO AND TOMATO SALAD WITH BASIL

Salad Description:

Avocado and Tomato Salad with Basil is a refreshing and vibrant dish celebrating the natural flavors of ripe avocados and juicy tomatoes. Enhanced with the aromatic freshness of basil, this salad has a simple yet elegant side that complements a variety of main courses.

Ingredients:

• Two ripe avocados, peeled, pitted, and diced

• 2 cups cherry tomatoes, halved

• 1/4 cup fresh basil leaves, chiffonade (thinly sliced)

• One tablespoon extra-virgin olive oil

• One tablespoon of balsamic vinegar

• Salt and pepper, to taste

• Optional: Feta cheese, crumbled, for garnish

Instructions:

Prepare Avocados and Tomatoes:

Peel, pit, and dice the ripe avocados. Halve the

cherry tomatoes.

Chiffonade Basil:

Stack the basil leaves and roll them into a tight bundle. Slice thinly across the roll to create chiffonade.

Combine Ingredients:

Gently combine the diced avocados, halved cherry tomatoes, and basil chiffonade in a large bowl.

Drizzle with Olive Oil and Balsamic Vinegar:

Drizzle extra-virgin olive oil and balsamic vinegar over the avocado and tomato mixture.

Season with Salt and Pepper:

Season the salad with salt and pepper according to your taste preference. Toss gently to coat the ingredients evenly.

Optional: Add Crumbled Feta:

If desired, sprinkle crumbled feta cheese over the salad for added creaminess and saltiness.

Serve Immediately:

Serve the Avocado and Tomato Salad with Basil immediately, allowing the fresh flavors to shine.

Serving Suggestions:

Pair with grilled chicken, shrimp, or fish for a light and nutritious meal.

Serve as a side dish at barbecues, picnics, or summer gatherings.

Enjoy on its own or atop a bed of mixed greens for a more substantial salad.

Nutrition Information (per serving, without feta):

- Calories: 200

- Protein: 3g

- Carbohydrates: 12g

- Fat: 17g

- Saturated Fat: 2.5g

- Cholesterol: 0mg

- Sodium: 10mg

- Fiber: 8g

- Sugar: 2g

BROCCOLI AND QUINOA STIR-FRY

Main Course Description:

Broccoli and Quinoa Stir-Fry is a wholesome and nutritious dish that combines broccoli's crunchiness with quinoa's protein-packed goodness. This stir-fry is flavored with a savory soy-ginger sauce, creating a satisfying and balanced meal that's quick and easy to prepare.

Ingredients:

For the Stir-Fry:

- 1 cup quinoa, rinsed
- 2 cups broccoli florets
- One red bell pepper, thinly sliced
- One carrot, julienned
- Three green onions, sliced
- One tablespoon of sesame oil
- 2 tablespoons vegetable oil
- Sesame seeds, for garnish (optional)

For the Sauce:

- Three tablespoons soy sauce

- One tablespoon of hoisin sauce

- One tablespoon of rice vinegar

- One tablespoon of honey or maple syrup

- One tablespoon of fresh ginger, minced

- 2 cloves garlic, minced

Instructions:

Cook Quinoa:

Combine 1 cup of rinsed quinoa in a medium saucepan with 2 cups of water. Bring to a boil, then reduce the heat, cover, and simmer for 15-20 minutes or until the quinoa is cooked and water is absorbed. Fluff with a fork.

Prepare Vegetables:

While the quinoa is cooking, prepare the vegetables. Cut the broccoli into small florets, thinly slice the red bell pepper, julienne the carrot, and slice the green onions.

Make the Sauce:

Whisk together soy sauce, hoisin sauce, rice vinegar, honey or maple syrup, minced ginger, and minced garlic in a small bowl. Set aside.

Stir-Fry Vegetables:

Heat vegetable oil in a large wok or skillet over medium-high heat. Add broccoli, red bell pepper, and julienned carrot. Stir-fry for 3-4 minutes or until the vegetables are slightly tender but still crisp.

Add Quinoa:

Add the cooked quinoa to the wok or skillet with the stir-fried vegetables. Mix well to combine.

Pour Sauce Over:

Pour the prepared sauce over the quinoa and vegetables. Toss to coat evenly.

Finish with Sesame Oil:

Drizzle sesame oil over the stir-fry and toss to incorporate the flavors.

Garnish and Serve:

Garnish with sliced green onions and sesame seeds (if using). Serve hot.

Serving Suggestions:

Top with grilled tofu, chicken, or shrimp for added protein.

Customize with your favorite stir-fry vegetables like snap peas or baby corn.

Drizzle with a bit of extra soy sauce or a squeeze of fresh lime before serving.

Nutrition Information (per serving):

- Calories: 400

- Protein: 12g

- Carbohydrates: 60g

- Fat: 14g

- Saturated Fat: 2g

- Cholesterol: 0mg

- Sodium: 600mg

- Fiber: 8g

- Sugar: 10g

LEMON-TURMERIC INFUSED WATER

Beverage Description:

Lemon-Turmeric Infused Water is a refreshing and healthful drink that combines lemon's citrusy brightness with turmeric's anti-inflammatory properties. This infused water quenches your thirst and provides a burst of flavor and potential health benefits.

Ingredients:

• One lemon, thinly sliced

• One teaspoon ground turmeric (or a small piece of fresh turmeric root)

• 1-2 tablespoons honey or agave syrup (optional for sweetness)

• Ice cubes

• Fresh mint leaves (optional, for garnish)

• 4 cups water

Instructions:

Prepare the Ingredients:

Wash the lemon thoroughly and slice it into thin rounds. If using fresh turmeric root, peel and cut it into thin pieces.

Infuse Water:

Combine the lemon slices and turmeric with 4 cups of water in a pitcher. Stir gently to release the flavors.

Sweeten (Optional):

Add honey or agave syrup to the water if you prefer a sweetened infusion. Adjust the sweetness to your liking and stir well to dissolve.

Chill:

Place the pitcher in the refrigerator and let the water infuse for 2-4 hours. For a more potent infusion, you can leave it overnight.

Serve Over Ice:

When ready to serve, add ice cubes to glasses and pour the lemon-turmeric infused water over the ice.

Garnish (Optional):

Garnish with fresh mint leaves for an extra burst of freshness and aroma.

Stir Before Serving:

Before serving, give the infused water a gentle stir to distribute the flavors evenly.

Enjoy:

Enjoy the Lemon-Turmeric Infused Water as a hydrating and flavorful beverage.

Tips:

• Experiment with the turmeric quantity to find your preferred level of spiciness.

• Adjust the sweetness to your taste preference by adding more or less honey or agave syrup.

• For a fizzy version, top off with sparkling water.

Health Benefits:

• Lemon: Rich in vitamin C, it supports digestion and adds a refreshing citrus flavor.

• Turmeric: Known for its anti-inflammatory and antioxidant properties.

• Honey or Agave Syrup: Provides natural sweetness and may offer additional health benefits.

GREEN TEA CHIA SEED PUDDING

Dessert or Breakfast Description:

Green Tea Chia Seed Pudding is a delightful and nutritious treat that combines green tea's earthy notes with the lovely texture of chia seeds. This pudding is a delicious dessert and makes for a satisfying and energizing breakfast option.

Ingredients:

For the Pudding:

- 1/4 cup chia seeds

- 1 cup almond milk (or any milk of your choice)

- One green tea bag

- One tablespoon of honey or maple syrup (adjust to taste)

- 1/2 teaspoon vanilla extract

For Topping:

- Sliced strawberries or kiwi

- Chopped nuts (almonds, pistachios, or your favorite)

- Fresh mint leaves for garnish

Instructions:

Brew Green Tea:

Steep the green tea bag in hot water according to the package instructions. Allow it to cool to room temperature.

Make Green Tea Base:

In a bowl, combine the brewed green tea with almond milk. Remove the green tea bag.

Sweeten and Flavor:

Add honey, maple syrup, and vanilla extract to the green tea and almond milk mixture. Stir well to combine.

Add Chia Seeds:

Sprinkle the chia seeds into the green tea mixture. Stir thoroughly to ensure the chia seeds are well distributed.

Refrigerate Overnight:

Cover the bowl and refrigerate the mixture for at least 4 hours or, ideally, overnight. This allows the chia seeds to absorb the liquid and create a pudding-like consistency.

Stir Before Serving:

Before serving, stir the pudding well to break up any clumps and achieve a smooth texture.

Serve with Toppings:

Spoon the Green Tea Chia Seed Pudding into serving bowls or jars. Top with sliced strawberries, kiwi, chopped nuts, and fresh mint leaves.

Enjoy:

Enjoy this delicious and nutrient-packed Green

Tea Chia Seed Pudding as a dessert or a healthy breakfast option.

Tips:

• Experiment with different flavors by adding matcha powder or a splash of coconut milk.

• Adjust the sweetness to your liking by adding more or less honey or maple syrup.

• Get creative with toppings – try coconut flakes, granola, or a drizzle of fruit compote.

Nutrition Information (per serving, without toppings):

• Calories: 200

• Protein: 5g

• Carbohydrates: 20g

• Fat: 12g

• Saturated Fat: 1g

• Cholesterol: 0mg

• Sodium: 80mg

• Fiber: 10g

• Sugar: 5g

CHIA SEED PUDDING WITH TURMERIC AND BERRIES

Dessert or Breakfast Description:

Chia Seed Pudding with Turmeric and Berries is a nutritious and vibrant dish that combines the superfood qualities of chia seeds with the anti-inflammatory benefits of turmeric and the sweetness of mixed berries. This pudding is a delightful dessert and a wholesome and satisfying breakfast option.

Ingredients:

For the Pudding:

• 1/4 cup chia seeds

• 1 cup coconut milk (or any milk of your choice)

• One teaspoon of ground turmeric

• One tablespoon of honey or maple syrup (adjust to taste)

• 1/2 teaspoon vanilla extract

For Topping:

• Mixed berries (strawberries, blueberries, raspberries)

- Sliced kiwi or banana
- Chopped nuts (almonds, walnuts)
- Coconut flakes
- Drizzle of honey or maple syrup

Instructions:

Prepare the Pudding Base:

Combine chia seeds, coconut milk, ground turmeric, honey or maple syrup, and vanilla extract in a bowl. Stir well to combine.

Mix Thoroughly:

Ensure that the chia seeds are evenly distributed in the mixture. Stir again after a few minutes to prevent clumping.

Refrigerate Overnight:

Cover the bowl and refrigerate the chia seed mixture for at least 4 hours or overnight. This allows the chia seeds to absorb the liquid and create a pudding-like consistency.

Stir Before Serving:

Before serving, stir the pudding well to achieve a smooth and consistent texture.

Layer with Berries and Toppings:

Layer the chia seed pudding with mixed berries, sliced kiwi or banana, and chopped nuts in serving jars or bowls.

Sprinkle Coconut Flakes:

Sprinkle coconut flakes over the top for added texture and flavor.

Drizzle with Honey or Maple Syrup:

Finish by drizzling a bit of honey or maple syrup over the layered chia seed pudding and berries.

Enjoy:

Enjoy this vibrant and nutrient-packed Chia Seed Pudding with Turmeric and Berries as a delicious dessert or a healthful breakfast.

Tips:

• Customize the pudding by adding your favorite spices like cinnamon or cardamom.

• Experiment with different types of milk for varied flavors – almond milk, soy milk, or dairy milk.

• Include a handful of granola for extra crunch and nutrition.

Nutrition Information (per serving):

• Calories: 250

• Protein: 6g

• Carbohydrates: 25g

• Fat: 15g

• Saturated Fat: 10g

• Cholesterol: 0mg

• Sodium: 20mg

• Fiber: 10g

• Sugar: 10g

DARK CHOCOLATE AND ALMOND ENERGY BITES

Snack Description:

Dark Chocolate and Almond Energy Bites are a delightful and nutritious snack that combines the rich flavors of dark chocolate with the crunch of almonds and the energy-boosting goodness of dates. These bite-sized treats are perfect for a quick pick-me-up during the day or as a satisfying pre-workout snack.

Ingredients:

- 1 cup almonds, raw and unsalted
- 1 cup pitted dates
- Two tablespoons cocoa powder (unsweetened)
- 1/4 cup dark chocolate chips (at least 70% cocoa)
- One teaspoon of vanilla extract
- Pinch of sea salt
- Shredded coconut or crushed almonds for coating (optional)

Instructions:

Prepare Almonds:

In a food processor, pulse the almonds until they are finely chopped. Be careful not to over-process; you want a slightly coarse texture for crunch.

Add Dates and Cocoa Powder:

Add the pitted dates, cocoa powder, dark chocolate chips, vanilla extract, and a pinch of sea salt to the chopped almonds in the food processor.

Blend Until Combined:

Process the mixture until it forms a sticky and uniform dough. You should be able to press the mixture together with your fingers.

Shape into Bites:

Roll small portions of the mixture between your palms to form bite-sized energy balls.

Coat with Coconut or Crushed Almonds (Optional):

Roll the energy bites in shredded coconut or crushed almonds for added texture and flavor.

Chill in the Refrigerator:

Place the energy bites on a tray or plate and refrigerate for at least 30 minutes to firm up.

Store in an Airtight Container:

Once firm, transfer the Dark Chocolate and Almond Energy Bites to an airtight container. Store in the refrigerator for a longer shelf life.

Enjoy:

Enjoy these delicious and nutritious energy bites as a quick snack or a pre-workout boost.

Tips:

• Customize the recipe by adding a tablespoon of nut butter for extra richness.

• Experiment with different coatings, such as crushed pistachios or chia seeds.

• Adjust sweetness by adding more dates if desired.

Nutrition Information (per serving, based on one energy bite):

• Calories: 80

• Protein: 2g

• Carbohydrates: 8g

• Fat: 5g

• Saturated Fat: 1g

• Cholesterol: 0mg

• Sodium: 5mg

• Fiber: 2g

• Sugar: 5g

AVOCADO CHOCOLATE MOUSSE

Dessert Description:

Avocado Chocolate Mousse is a decadent and creamy dessert that combines the richness of ripe avocados with the indulgence of dark chocolate. This luscious mousse is delicious and a healthier alternative, as avocados provide a velvety texture without the need for heavy cream.

Ingredients:

• Two ripe avocados, peeled and pitted

• 1/2 cup unsweetened cocoa powder

• 1/2 cup maple syrup or honey (adjust to taste)

• 1/4 cup almond milk or any milk of your choice

• One teaspoon of vanilla extract

• A pinch of salt

• Dark chocolate shavings or grated chocolate for garnish (optional)

• Fresh berries or mint leaves for topping (optional)

Instructions:

Prepare Avocados:

Ensure the avocados are ripe, and scoop out the flesh from both avocados.

Blend Ingredients:

Combine the avocado flesh, cocoa powder, maple syrup or honey, almond milk, vanilla extract, and a pinch of salt in a food processor or blender.

Blend Until Smooth:

Blend the ingredients until the mixture becomes smooth and velvety. Scrape down the sides of the blender or food processor as needed to ensure even mixing.

Taste and Adjust:

Taste the chocolate mousse and adjust the sweetness if needed by adding more maple syrup or honey.

Chill in the Refrigerator:

Transfer the chocolate mousse into serving bowls or glasses and refrigerate for at least 2 hours to allow it to set.

Garnish Before Serving:

Before serving, garnish the Avocado Chocolate Mousse with dark chocolate shavings or grated chocolate. Top with fresh berries or mint leaves if desired.

Serve Chilled:

Serve the chilled Avocado Chocolate Mousse for a delightful and guilt-free dessert experience.

Tips:

• For a more intense chocolate flavor, use dark cocoa powder.

• Experiment with toppings such as chopped nuts, coconut flakes, or a dollop of whipped cream.

• Adjust the consistency by adding more milk if you prefer a lighter mousse.

Nutrition Information (per serving):

• Calories: 200

• Protein: 3g

• Carbohydrates: 25g

• Fat: 12g

• Saturated Fat: 3g

• Cholesterol: 0mg

• Sodium: 20mg

• Fiber: 7g

• Sugar: 14g

ROASTED TURMERIC CHICKPEAS

Snack Description:

Roasted Turmeric Chickpeas are a crunchy and flavorful snack that combines the nuttiness of chickpeas with the warm, earthy notes of turmeric. This simple and nutritious snack is not only addictive but also packed with protein and fiber, making it a satisfying option for on-the-go munching.

Ingredients:

• Two cans (15 ounces each) of chickpeas, drained and rinsed

• 2 tablespoons olive oil

• One teaspoon of ground turmeric

• 1/2 teaspoon ground cumin

• 1/2 teaspoon smoked paprika

• 1/4 teaspoon cayenne pepper (adjust to taste)

• Salt, to taste

• Freshly ground black pepper, to taste

Instructions:

Preheat the Oven:

Preheat your oven to 400°F (200°C).

Dry Chickpeas:

Pat the rinsed chickpeas dry using a clean kitchen towel or paper towels. Removing excess moisture helps in achieving crispiness.

Combine Ingredients:

Toss the dried chickpeas in a bowl with olive oil, ground turmeric, ground cumin, smoked paprika, cayenne pepper, salt, and freshly ground black pepper. Ensure that the chickpeas are evenly coated with the spice mixture.

Spread on Baking Sheet:

Spread the seasoned chickpeas in a single layer on a baking sheet lined with parchment paper.

Roast in the Oven:

Roast the chickpeas in the preheated oven for 25-30 minutes or until they are golden brown and crispy. Shake the pan or stir the chickpeas halfway through the baking time for even cooking.

Cool Before Serving:

Allow the roasted turmeric chickpeas to cool on the baking sheet before transferring them to a serving bowl. They will continue to crisp up as they cool.

Serve and Enjoy:

Serve the Roasted Turmeric Chickpeas as a tasty and nutritious snack. Enjoy them on their own or as a crunchy topping for salads.

Tips:

• Customize the spice blend by adding your favorite herbs or spices.

• Store the roasted chickpeas in an airtight container for up to a week.

• Experiment with different levels of cayenne pepper to control the spiciness.

Nutrition Information (per serving):

• Calories: 150

• Protein: 6g

• Carbohydrates: 21g

• Fat: 5g

• Saturated Fat: 0.5g

• Cholesterol: 0mg

• Sodium: 300mg

• Fiber: 6g

• Sugar: 1g

KALE CHIPS WITH OLIVE OIL AND SEA SALT

Snack Description:

Kale Chips with Olive Oil and Sea Salt are a crispy and flavorful snack that transforms kale into a delicious and nutritious treat. This simple recipe highlights the natural goodness of kale while enhancing its texture with a touch of olive oil and a sprinkle of sea salt. Enjoy these guilt-free chips as a wholesome alternative to traditional potato chips.

Ingredients:

• One bunch of kale stems was removed and leaves were torn into bite-sized pieces

• 2 tablespoons olive oil

• Sea salt, to taste

Instructions:

Preheat the Oven:

Preheat your oven to 350°F (175°C).

Clean and Dry Kale:

Wash the kale leaves thoroughly and ensure they

are scorched. You can use a salad spinner or pat them dry with a clean kitchen towel.

Remove Stems and Tear into Pieces:

Remove the tough stems from the kale leaves and tear the remaining leaves into bite-sized pieces.

Massage with Olive Oil:

In a large bowl, drizzle the torn kale leaves with olive oil. Handly massage the oil into the kale leaves, ensuring each piece is lightly coated.

Spread on Baking Sheet:

Arrange the kale pieces in a single layer on a baking sheet lined with parchment paper. Make sure they are not overcrowded to allow for even crisping.

Sprinkle with Sea Salt:

Sprinkle sea salt over the kale pieces. The amount of salt can be adjusted according to your taste preference.

Bake in the Oven:

Bake in the preheated oven for 10-15 minutes or until the edges of the kale are crisp and lightly browned. Keep a close eye to prevent burning.

Cool Before Serving:

Allow the Kale Chips to cool on the baking sheet for a few minutes. They will continue to crisp up as they cool.

Serve and Enjoy:

Transfer the Kale Chips to a bowl and enjoy them as a crunchy and nutritious snack.

Tips:

• For extra flavor, experiment with additional seasonings such as garlic powder, nutritional yeast, or chili flakes.

• Rotate the baking sheet halfway through the cooking time to ensure even crisping.

• Store any leftovers in an airtight container to maintain crispness.

Nutrition Information (per serving):

• Calories: 80

• Protein: 3g

• Carbohydrates: 6g

• Fat: 6g

• Saturated Fat: 1g

• Cholesterol: 0mg

• Sodium: 150mg

• Fiber: 2g

• Sugar: 0g

CHAPTER FOUR

Hydration-Focused Recipes

Cucumber and Mint Infused Water

Beverage Description:

Cucumber and Mint Infused Water is a refreshing and hydrating beverage that adds a burst of flavor to plain Water. This infused Water is delicious and provides a cooling sensation, making it the perfect choice for staying hydrated on warm days. It's a simple and healthy alternative to sugary drinks.

Ingredients:

• 1/2 cucumber, thinly sliced

• 1/4 cup fresh mint leaves

• Ice cubes

• 4 cups Water

Instructions:

Prepare Ingredients:

Wash the cucumber thoroughly and slice it into thin rounds. Rinse the fresh mint leaves.

Combine Cucumber and Mint:

In a pitcher, combine the cucumber slices and fresh mint leaves.

Muddle Mint (Optional):

If you prefer a more robust mint flavor, gently muddle the mint leaves in the pitcher using a wooden spoon or muddler. This helps release the mint's essential oils.

Add Ice Cubes:

Place ice cubes over the cucumber and mint mixture. This will keep the infused Water cool.

Pour Water:

Pour 4 cups of Water into the pitcher, covering the cucumber and mint.

Stir Gently:

Give the ingredients a gentle stir to distribute the flavors.

Refrigerate:

Place the pitcher in the refrigerator and let the Water infuse for at least 1-2 hours. You can leave it in the fridge overnight for a more intense flavor.

Serve Chilled:

When ready to serve, pour the Cucumber and Mint Infused Water into glasses, ensuring some cucumber slices and mint leaves are included.

Garnish (Optional):

Garnish each glass with a cucumber slice or a sprig of fresh mint for a decorative touch.

Enjoy:

Sip and enjoy the refreshing taste of Cucumber and Mint Infused Water as a healthy and hydrating beverage.

Tips:

• For variation, add a few lemon slices for a citrusy twist.

• Adjust the intensity of flavors by adding more cucumber or mint according to your preference.

• Replenish the Water in the pitcher throughout the day

for a continuous infusion.

Health Benefits:

• Cucumber: Hydrating and contains vitamins and minerals.

• Mint: Refreshing, aids digestion, and adds a pleasant aroma.

• Hydration: Promotes water intake with a burst of natural flavors.

This Cucumber and Mint Infused Water is a delightful and healthy way to stay hydrated, especially when you want a break from plain Water. The combination of cool cucumber and invigorating mint creates a refreshing drink that's perfect for any occasion. Enjoy the natural flavors while reaping the benefits of staying well-hydrated.

COCONUT WATER SMOOTHIE WITH PINEAPPLE

Smoothie Description:

The Coconut Water Smoothie with Pineapple is a tropical and hydrating blend that combines the natural sweetness of pineapple with the refreshing taste of coconut water. Packed with vitamins, minerals, and electrolytes, this smoothie is delicious and a revitalizing choice to keep you energized.

Ingredients:

• 1 cup coconut water

• 1 cup fresh or frozen pineapple chunks

• 1/2 banana (fresh or frozen)

• 1/2 cup Greek yogurt or coconut yogurt

• Handful of ice cubes

• Optional: 1 tablespoon chia seeds or flaxseeds for added nutrition

• Optional: Honey or agave syrup to sweeten (adjust to taste)

Instructions:

Prepare Ingredients:

If using fresh pineapple, peel and cut it into chunks. If using a fresh banana, peel and slice it.

Combine in Blender:

Combine coconut water, pineapple chunks, banana, Greek yogurt, or coconut yogurt, and ice cubes in a blender.

Add Optional Ingredients:

If desired, add chia seeds or flaxseeds for added fiber and omega-3 fatty acids.

Blend Until Smooth:

Blend the ingredients on high speed until the mixture becomes smooth and creamy.

Taste and Sweeten (Optional):

Taste the smoothie and, if needed, add honey or agave syrup to sweeten. Blend again to incorporate.

Pour and Serve:

Pour the Coconut Water Smoothie with Pineapple into glasses.

Garnish (Optional):

Garnish with a slice of pineapple on the rim of the glass or a wedge for a decorative touch.

Enjoy:

Sip and enjoy this tropical and hydrating smoothie as a delicious and nutritious beverage.

Tips:

• For a thicker consistency, use frozen pineapple and banana.

• Customize by adding spinach or kale for a green boost.

• Experiment with other tropical fruits like mango or kiwi for varied flavors.

Nutrition Information (per serving):

• Calories: 150

• Protein: 5g

• Carbohydrates: 30g

• Fat: 2g

• Saturated Fat: 1g

• Cholesterol: 0mg

• Sodium: 60mg

• Fiber: 4g

• Sugar: 20g

CHAMOMILE, PEPPERMINT, OR GINGER HERBAL TEA

Tea Description:

Chamomile, Peppermint, or Ginger Herbal Tea is a soothing and aromatic beverage offering various health benefits. Whether you choose the calming notes of chamomile, the invigorating freshness of peppermint, or the warming spice of ginger, each herbal tea variant provides a delightful and comforting experience.

Ingredients:

For Chamomile Tea:

• One chamomile tea bag or one tablespoon of dried chamomile flowers

• 1 cup hot Water

• Optional: Honey or lemon for sweetness

For Peppermint Tea:

• One peppermint tea bag or one tablespoon of dried peppermint leaves

• 1 cup hot Water

• Optional: Honey or a mint sprig for added flavor

For Ginger Tea:

• 1-inch piece of fresh ginger, thinly sliced

• 1 cup hot Water

• Optional: Honey or lemon for sweetness

Instructions:

For Chamomile Tea:

1. Place a chamomile tea bag or dried chamomile flowers in a cup.

2. Pour hot Water over the chamomile.

3. Allow it to steep for 5-7 minutes.

4. Optionally, add honey or a squeeze of lemon for sweetness.

5. Remove the tea bag or strain the chamomile flowers.

6. Enjoy the calming and mild flavor of Chamomile Tea.

For Peppermint Tea:

1. Place a peppermint tea bag or dried peppermint leaves in a cup.

2. Pour hot Water over the peppermint.

3. Let it steep for 5-7 minutes.

4. Optionally, add honey or a fresh mint sprig for extra flavor.

5. Remove the tea bag or strain the peppermint leaves.

6. Savor the refreshing and minty taste of Peppermint Tea.

For Ginger Tea:

1. Place thinly sliced fresh ginger in a cup.

2. Pour hot Water over the ginger.

3. Allow it to steep for 5-10 minutes, depending on desired strength.

4. Optionally, add honey or a squeeze of lemon for sweetness.

5. Strain the ginger slices.

6. Enjoy the warming and spicy notes of Ginger Tea.

Tips:

• Adjust the steeping time based on your preference for a firmer or milder flavor.

• Experiment with combinations like chamomile and ginger for a unique blend.

• Enhance the experience by enjoying your tea in a cozy setting.

Health Benefits:

• Chamomile Tea: Calming, may aid in sleep, and has anti-inflammatory properties.

• Peppermint Tea: Aids digestion, relieves headaches, and provides a refreshing flavor.

• Ginger Tea: Supports digestion, helps with nausea, and adds a warming sensation.

These herbal teas—Chamomile, Peppermint, or Ginger—are delicious and offer a range of potential health benefits. Whether you seek relaxation, freshness, or warmth, each variant provides a delightful and comforting way to enjoy herbal infusions. Sip mindfully

and savor the soothing qualities of your chosen herbal
tea.

WATERMELON MINT SALAD

Salad Description:

Watermelon Mint Salad is a refreshing and hydrating dish that combines juicy watermelon's sweetness with fresh mint's refreshing flavor. This vibrant salad is perfect for hot summer days or as a side dish to complement a variety of meals. It's a simple yet delightful way to enjoy the natural goodness of seasonal fruits.

Ingredients:

• 4 cups cubed seedless watermelon

• 1/2 cup fresh mint leaves, thinly sliced or torn

• 1/2 cup feta cheese, crumbled (optional)

• One tablespoon extra-virgin olive oil

• One tablespoon of balsamic glaze or aged balsamic vinegar

• Pinch of salt

• Optional: Black pepper for a hint of spice

Instructions:

Prepare Watermelon:

Cut the watermelon into bite-sized cubes, removing seeds if present. Place the cubed watermelon in a large mixing bowl.

Add Fresh Mint:

Wash and thinly slice or tear the fresh mint leaves. Add them to the bowl with the watermelon.

Optional: Crumble Feta:

If using feta cheese, crumble it over the watermelon and mint. Feta adds a salty and creamy contrast to the sweetness of the watermelon.

Drizzle with Olive Oil:

Drizzle extra-virgin olive oil over the salad. This enhances the flavors and adds a subtle richness.

Drizzle with Balsamic Glaze:

Drizzle balsamic glaze or aged balsamic vinegar over the salad for a sweet and tangy finish.

Season with Salt:

Sprinkle a pinch of salt over the salad to balance the sweetness and enhance the overall taste.

Optional: Add Black Pepper:

You can add freshly ground black pepper to taste for a hint of spice.

Gently Toss:

Gently toss the ingredients together to ensure an even coating of the olive oil, balsamic glaze, and seasonings.

Chill (Optional):

If desired, refrigerate the Watermelon Mint Salad for about 15-30 minutes before serving for a refreshing chill.

Serve:

Transfer the salad to a serving platter or individual bowls and serve immediately.

Tips:

• Choose ripe and sweet watermelon for the best flavor.

• Adjust the quantity of mint, olive oil, and balsamic glaze to suit your taste preferences.

• Experiment with additional ingredients like cucumber or arugula for added freshness.

Nutrition Information (per serving, without feta):

• Calories: 80

• Protein: 1g

• Carbohydrates: 20g

• Fat: 1g

• Saturated Fat: 0g

• Cholesterol: 0mg

• Sodium: 50mg

• Fiber: 1g

• Sugar: 17g

CUCUMBER-LEMON DETOX WATER

Detox Water Description:

Cucumber-Lemon Detox Water is a refreshing and hydrating beverage infused with the natural detoxifying properties of cucumber and the zesty freshness of lemon. This simple detox water is delicious, helps promote hydration, and supports your body's biological cleansing processes.

Ingredients:

• 1/2 cucumber, thinly sliced

• 1/2 lemon, thinly sliced

• 4 cups cold Water

• Ice cubes

• Optional: Fresh mint leaves for added flavor

• Optional: A pinch of cayenne pepper for a metabolism boost

Instructions:

Prepare Ingredients:

Wash the cucumber and lemon thoroughly. Slice them into thin rounds or wedges.

Combine in a Pitcher:

In a large pitcher, combine the thinly sliced cucumber and lemon.

Add Optional Ingredients:

If desired, add a handful of fresh mint leaves for added freshness. For a metabolism boost, add a pinch of cayenne pepper.

Pour Cold Water:

Pour 4 cups of cold Water over the ingredients. Ensure that the cucumber and lemon slices are fully immersed.

Stir Gently:

Give the ingredients a gentle stir to distribute the flavors.

Add Ice Cubes:

Drop in a few ice cubes to keep the detox water cool.

Refrigerate:

Place the pitcher in the refrigerator and let the detox water infuse for at least 2 hours, or preferably overnight.

Serve Chilled:

When ready to serve, pour the Cucumber-Lemon Detox Water into glasses, making sure to include some cucumber and lemon slices.

Optional: Strain (If Preferred):

You can strain the detox water before serving if you prefer a smoother texture.

Enjoy:

Sip and enjoy this refreshing and hydrating Cucumber-Lemon Detox Water as a healthy beverage.

Tips:

• Adjust the intensity of flavors by adding more or fewer cucumber and lemon slices.

• Experiment with variations like adding ginger slices for an extra kick.

• Refill the pitcher with Water throughout the day for continuous hydration.

Health Benefits:

• Cucumber: Hydrating, contains antioxidants, and may support skin health.

• Lemon: Rich in vitamin C, it aids digestion and adds a refreshing taste.

• Mint: Adds a burst of freshness and may help with digestion.

• Cayenne Pepper May boost metabolism and add a subtle heat.

This Cucumber-Lemon Detox Water is a simple and effective way to stay hydrated while enjoying the infused ingredients' natural flavors and potential health benefits. Whether you're looking for a refreshing drink or a gentle detox option, this beverage is delightful. Sip mindfully and embrace the hydrating goodness of this detox water.

BERRY AND SPINACH SMOOTHIE

Smoothie Description:

The Berry and Spinach Smoothie is a delicious and nutrient-packed beverage that combines the sweetness of mixed berries with the vibrant goodness of spinach. Packed with vitamins, antioxidants, and fiber, this smoothie is tasty and a healthy addition to your day.

Ingredients:

• 1 cup mixed berries (strawberries, blueberries, raspberries)

• 1 cup fresh spinach leaves, washed

• 1/2 banana (fresh or frozen)

• 1/2 cup Greek yogurt or dairy-free alternative

• 1/2 cup almond milk or any milk of your choice

• One tablespoon of chia seeds (optional)

• Ice cubes

Instructions:

Prepare Ingredients:

Wash the berries and spinach leaves thoroughly. If using fresh berries, hull the strawberries.

Combine in Blender:

Combine the mixed berries, fresh spinach leaves, banana, Greek yogurt, almond milk, and chia seeds in a blender.

Add Ice Cubes:

Drop in a handful of ice cubes to make the smoothie chilled and refreshing.

Blend Until Smooth:

Blend the ingredients on high speed until the mixture becomes smooth and creamy.

Adjust Consistency:

If the smoothie is too thick, add more almond milk in small amounts until you reach your desired consistency.

Pour into Glasses:

Pour the Berry and Spinach Smoothie into glasses.

Optional: Garnish:

Optionally, garnish with a few whole berries or a sprinkle of chia seeds for a decorative touch.

Enjoy:

Sip and enjoy this vibrant and nutrient-rich Berry and Spinach Smoothie as a refreshing and healthy beverage.

Tips:

• Use frozen berries for a colder and thicker smoothie.

- Customize with additional ingredients like a tablespoon of honey or a scoop of protein powder.

- Experiment with different greens, such as kale or arugula, for variety.

Nutrition Information (per serving):

- Calories: 150

- Protein: 7g

- Carbohydrates: 25g

- Fat: 3g

- Saturated Fat: 0.5g

- Cholesterol: 0mg

- Sodium: 70mg

- Fiber: 7g

- Sugar: 15g

HYDRATING GREEN TEA MATCHA LATTE

Matcha Latte Description:

The Hydrating Green Tea Matcha Latte is a refreshing and energizing beverage that combines matcha's rich, earthy flavor with the creamy goodness of milk. Packed with antioxidants and known for its hydrating properties, this latte is a delightful way to enjoy the benefits of green tea in a creamy and comforting form.

Ingredients:

• One teaspoon of matcha powder

• 1 cup hot water (not boiling)

• 1/2 cup unsweetened almond milk or any milk of your choice

• One tablespoon of honey or sweetener of your choice (adjust to taste)

• Ice cubes (optional)

Instructions:

Prepare Matcha:

In a bowl, sift the matcha powder to remove any lumps.

Whisk Matcha:

Add a small amount of hot Water to the matcha powder to create a smooth paste. Use a bamboo or small whisk to blend until no lumps remain.

Add Hot Water:

Pour the remaining hot Water into the bowl with the matcha paste. Whisk briskly in a "W" or "M" shape motion until frothy.

Heat Milk:

Heat the almond milk in a separate saucepan or using a milk frother until it's warm but not boiling.

Combine Matcha and Milk:

Pour the frothy matcha over the warm almond milk. Mix gently to combine.

Sweeten to Taste:

Add honey or your preferred sweetener to the matcha latte. Adjust the sweetness to your liking.

Optional: Add Ice Cubes:

Add ice cubes to the drink if you prefer a cold matcha latte.

Stir and Enjoy:

Stir the matcha latte well and sip on this hydrating and delightful beverage.

Tips:

• Use a matcha bowl and whisk for an authentic preparation.

• Experiment with different milk alternatives like coconut or soy milk.

• Try incorporating a dash of vanilla extract or a sprinkle

of cinnamon for added flavor.

Nutrition Information (per serving):

- Calories: 50
- Protein: 1g
- Carbohydrates: 12g
- Fat: 0.5g
- Saturated Fat: 0g
- Cholesterol: 0mg
- Sodium: 80mg
- Fiber: 1g
- Sugar: 10g

HOMEMADE ELECTROLYTE DRINK WITH COCONUT WATER

Electrolyte Drink Description:

This Homemade Electrolyte Drink with Coconut Water is a natural and refreshing beverage that helps replenish electrolytes lost during physical activity or dehydration. Coconut water serves as a hydrating base, while added ingredients provide essential minerals and a hint of natural sweetness.

Ingredients:

• 2 cups coconut water

• 1/2 cup orange juice (freshly squeezed)

• One tablespoon of honey or maple syrup

• 1/4 teaspoon sea salt

• 1/4 teaspoon baking soda

• Ice cubes (optional)

Instructions:

Gather Ingredients:

Ensure you have fresh coconut water, orange juice, honey or maple syrup, sea salt, and baking soda.

Mix Coconut Water and Orange Juice:

In a pitcher, combine the coconut water and freshly squeezed orange juice.

Add Sweetener:

Add honey or maple syrup to the mixture. Adjust the sweetness according to your preference.

Include Sea Salt:

Incorporate sea salt into the mixture. Sea salt provides sodium, an essential electrolyte.

Add Baking Soda:

Add a small amount of baking soda. Baking soda contains sodium and helps balance the pH levels.

Stir Thoroughly:

Stir the ingredients thoroughly to ensure that the sweetener, salt, and baking soda are well-distributed.

Optional: Add Ice Cubes:

Add ice cubes to the pitcher if you prefer a chilled electrolyte drink.

Refrigerate:

Place the pitcher in the refrigerator for at least 30 minutes to allow the flavors to meld and the drink to chill.

Stir Before Serving:

Before serving, give the electrolyte drink a final stir to make sure all ingredients are well-mixed.

Serve and Hydrate:

Pour the Homemade Electrolyte Drink into glasses and enjoy this natural and hydrating beverage.

Tips:

• Use freshly squeezed orange juice for the best flavor and nutritional content.

• Adjust the sweetness, salt, and baking soda quantities to suit your taste preferences.

• Experiment with different citrus juices for varied flavors.

Nutrition Information (per serving):

• Calories: 70

• Protein: 1g

• Carbohydrates: 18g

• Fat: 0g

• Saturated Fat: 0g

• Cholesterol: 0mg

• Sodium: 300mg

• Fiber: 0g

• Sugar: 15g

ORANGE AND BASIL-INFUSED WATER

Infused Water Description:

Orange and Basil Infused Water is a refreshing and flavorful beverage that combines the citrusy sweetness of oranges with the herbal notes of fresh basil. This naturally infused Water adds a burst of taste and provides a hydrating and healthful option without added sugars or artificial flavors.

Ingredients:

• One orange, thinly sliced

• 5-6 fresh basil leaves

• 1 liter (4 cups) cold water

• Ice cubes (optional)

Instructions:

Prepare Ingredients:

Wash the orange thoroughly and thinly slice it, including the peel, for added flavor. Rinse the fresh basil leaves.

Combine in a Pitcher:

In a large pitcher, combine the sliced orange and fresh basil leaves.

Muddle Basil (Optional):

For a more pronounced basil flavor, gently muddle the basil leaves in the pitcher using a wooden spoon or muddler.

Add Cold Water:

Pour 1 liter (4 cups) of cold Water into the pitcher over the orange and basil.

Optional: Add Ice Cubes:

If you prefer a chilled infusion, add ice cubes to the pitcher.

Stir Gently:

Give the ingredients a gentle stir to distribute the flavors.

Refrigerate:

Place the pitcher in the refrigerator and let the Orange and Basil Infused Water chill for at least 2 hours, or preferably overnight, to allow the flavors to infuse.

Serve and Enjoy:

When ready to serve, pour the infused Water into glasses, ensuring each serving has orange slices and basil leaves.

Tips:

• Experiment with variations by adding other herbs like mint or rosemary.

• Squeeze a little juice from the orange slices into the

Water for extra citrus flavor.

• Refill the pitcher with Water throughout the day to continue enjoying the infused flavors.

Health Benefits:

• Oranges: Rich in vitamin C and antioxidants, support immune health.

• Basil: It contains antioxidants, may have anti-inflammatory properties, and adds a fresh herbal flavor.

This Orange and Basil Infused Water is a delightful and hydrating option, perfect for those looking to enjoy a refreshing drink without added sugars or artificial ingredients. The combination of orange and basil creates a harmonious and flavorful infusion that makes staying hydrated a more enjoyable experience. Sip and savor the natural goodness of this citrusy and herbal blend.

ALOE VERA JUICE WITH FRESH LIME

Juice Description:

Aloe Vera Juice with Fresh Lime is a rejuvenating and hydrating beverage that combines the soothing properties of aloe vera with the zesty citrus kick of fresh lime. This refreshing drink offers a burst of flavor and potential health benefits, making it a delightful addition to your wellness routine.

Ingredients:

• 1/2 cup pure aloe vera juice (without added sugars)

• Juice of 1 fresh lime

• One tablespoon of honey or agave syrup (optional for sweetness)

• 1 cup cold Water

• Ice cubes

Instructions:

Prepare Aloe Vera Juice:

Ensure you have pure aloe vera juice without added sugars or flavorings.

Juice Fresh Lime:

Squeeze the juice of one fresh lime into a bowl,

removing any seeds.

Combine Aloe Vera Juice and Lime Juice:

Combine the aloe vera juice and fresh lime juice in a glass or pitcher.

Add Sweetener (Optional):

Add honey or agave syrup to the mixture if you prefer a sweeter taste. Adjust the sweetness to your liking.

Pour Cold Water:

Pour 1 cup of cold Water into the glass or pitcher.

Stir Thoroughly:

Stir the ingredients thoroughly to ensure the aloe vera, lime, and sweeteners are well mixed.

Add Ice Cubes:

Drop in a few ice cubes to keep the drink chilled.

Stir Again Before Serving:

Before serving, give the Aloe Vera Juice with Fresh Lime a final stir to make sure all ingredients are well-distributed.

Serve and Enjoy:

Pour the refreshing Aloe Vera Juice with Fresh Lime into a glass and savor the refreshing flavors.

Tips:

• Choose aloe vera juice that is specifically intended for consumption and free from additives.

• Adjust the lime juice and sweetener quantities based on your taste preferences.

• Garnish with a slice of lime for a decorative touch.

Health Benefits:

• Aloe Vera: Known for its potential anti-inflammatory and digestive benefits.

• Lime: Rich in vitamin C, it adds a zesty flavor and may support immune health.

WATERMELON CUBES WITH FRESH MINT

Refreshing Summer Snack Description: Watermelon Cubes with Fresh Mint is a simple and hydrating summer snack that combines the natural sweetness of juicy watermelon with the excellent aromatic notes of fresh mint. This delightful pairing satisfies your sweet cravings and provides a burst of refreshment on warm days.

Ingredients:

• 4 cups watermelon, cut into bite-sized cubes

• Fresh mint leaves, finely chopped or torn

• Optional: Lime wedges for extra citrusy flavor

Instructions:

Prepare Watermelon:

Wash and peel a ripe watermelon. Cut it into bite-sized cubes, removing seeds if necessary.

Chop Fresh Mint:

Wash the fresh mint leaves and either finely chop or tear them into smaller pieces.

Combine Watermelon and Mint:

In a large bowl, combine the watermelon cubes with the chopped or torn fresh mint.

Toss Gently:

Toss the watermelon and mint together gently to ensure an even distribution of flavors.

Optional: Add Lime Wedges:

For an extra citrusy kick, serve the Watermelon Cubes with Fresh Mint with lime wedges on the side. Squeeze lime juice over the watermelon before eating.

Chill (Optional):

If desired, refrigerate the watermelon cubes for about 15-30 minutes before serving for a refreshing chill.

Serve and Enjoy:

Plate the Watermelon Cubes with Fresh Mint and lime wedges, if used. Enjoy this hydrating and delightful summer snack.

Tips:

• Choose a seedless watermelon for convenience.

• Experiment with other herbs like basil for a different flavor profile.

• Customize by adding a sprinkle of chili powder for a sweet and spicy twist.

Nutrition Information (per serving):

• Calories: 50

• Protein: 1g

- Carbohydrates: 13g
- Fat: 0g
- Saturated Fat: 0g
- Cholesterol: 0mg
- Sodium: 2mg
- Fiber: 1g
- Sugar: 9g

GREEN TEA ICE POPS

Refreshing Summer Treat Description:

Green Tea Ice Pops are a cool and refreshing summer treat that combines the antioxidant-rich goodness of green tea with a hint of natural sweetness. These ice pops are a delightful way to stay calm and provide a unique and healthful twist to your frozen treats.

Ingredients:

• 2 cups brewed green tea, cooled

• 1-2 tablespoons honey or agave syrup (adjust to taste)

• 1/2 teaspoon pure vanilla extract (optional)

• Fresh mint leaves, finely chopped (optional)

• Sliced strawberries or kiwi (optional for added freshness)

Instructions:

Brew Green Tea:

Brew 2 cups of green tea and allow it to cool to room temperature.

Sweeten the Tea:

Once the green tea has cooled, add honey or agave syrup to sweeten. Adjust the sweetness according to your taste preferences.

Add Vanilla Extract (Optional):

Optionally, add pure vanilla extract to enhance the flavor. Stir well to combine.

Chop Fresh Mint (Optional):

Finely chop the leaves and add them to the sweetened green tea if using fresh mint. This adds a refreshing herbal note.

Prepare Ice Pop Molds:

If your ice pop molds have slots for fruit, add a few slices of strawberries or kiwi to each mold for added freshness and visual appeal.

Pour Green Tea Mixture:

Pour the sweetened green tea (with or without mint) into the ice pop molds, covering the fruit slices if added.

Insert Sticks:

Place the ice pop sticks into the molds. If your molds have lids, secure them to keep the sticks in place.

Freeze:

Place the ice pop molds in the freezer and let them freeze for at least 4-6 hours or until completely solid.

Unmold and Enjoy:

Once frozen, remove the Green Tea Ice Pops from the molds. If they're challenging to remove, briefly run the molds under warm Water to loosen the pops.

Serve and Garnish (Optional):

Serve the Green Tea Ice Pops on a hot day. Garnish with additional fresh mint leaves for a decorative touch.

Tips:

• For a floral twist, experiment with different tea varieties, like jasmine green tea.

• Add a splash of lemon or lime juice for a citrusy kick.

• Customize with your favorite fruits or herbs for a personalized touch.

Nutrition Information (per ice pop):

• Calories: 20

• Protein: 0g

• Carbohydrates: 5g

• Fat: 0g

• Saturated Fat: 0g

• Cholesterol: 0mg

• Sodium: 0mg

• Fiber: 0g

• Sugar: 4g

COCONUT WATER AND PINEAPPLE ICE CUBES

Tropical Ice Cube Description:

Coconut Water and Pineapple Ice Cubes are a refreshing and tropical twist to regular ice cubes. These flavored ice cubes add a burst of natural sweetness to your beverages and are perfect for cooling down on hot days. Use them in Water, iced tea, or your favorite tropical cocktails.

Ingredients:

• 2 cups coconut water

• 1 cup fresh pineapple juice (from about 1 cup of pineapple chunks)

• Pineapple chunks (optional for visual appeal)

Instructions:

Prepare Coconut Water:

Measure 2 cups of coconut water. Use fresh coconut water for the best flavor.

Extract Pineapple Juice:

Suppose you use fresh pineapple; peel and core the pineapple. Blend the pineapple chunks until smooth, then strain the juice to remove any pulp. Measure 1 cup of fresh pineapple juice.

Combine Coconut Water and Pineapple Juice:

Combine coconut water and fresh pineapple juice in a mixing bowl or jug. Stir well to ensure even distribution.

Prepare Ice Cube Trays:

If desired, place a small pineapple chunk in each ice cube tray compartment for added visual appeal.

Pour Mixture into Ice Cube Trays:

Carefully pour the coconut water and pineapple juice mixture into the ice cube trays, covering the pineapple chunks if added.

Freeze:

Place the ice cube trays in the freezer and let them freeze for at least 4-6 hours or until fully solid.

Remove from Trays:

Once frozen, remove the Coconut Water and Pineapple Ice Cubes from the trays. If they're sticking, you can loosen the tray's bottom under warm Water.

Store in a Freezer Bag (Optional):

Transfer the ice cubes to a freezer bag for easy storage. This prevents them from absorbing other freezer odors.

Use in Beverages:

Drop these tropical ice cubes into your favorite beverages to add a refreshing and sweet twist.

They're great in Water, iced tea, or tropical cocktails.

Tips:

• Use silicone ice cube trays for easy removal.

• Experiment with different fruit juices like mango or passion fruit for variety.

• Store the flavored ice cubes in a separate bag to maintain their freshness.

Enjoy the Tropical Twist:

Coconut Water and Pineapple Ice Cubes are a delightful way to infuse a tropical essence into your drinks. Whether you're sipping on Water or enjoying a summer cocktail, these ice cubes bring a burst of natural sweetness and a hint of the tropics to your beverage experience. Cool down and enjoy the refreshing vibes of these tropical ice cubes!

INFUSED WATERMELON SKEWERS

Refreshing Fruit Skewers Description:

Infused Watermelon Skewers are a creative and refreshing way to elevate the presentation of watermelon. These skewers are infused with the flavors of mint and lime, adding a burst of freshness to the natural sweetness of the watermelon. Serve them as a colorful and hydrating snack at picnics and parties or as a delightful treat on hot days.

Ingredients:

- Watermelon, seedless, cut into bite-sized cubes

- Fresh mint leaves

- Limes, sliced into thin rounds

- Wooden or bamboo skewers

Instructions:

Prepare Watermelon:

Wash the watermelon and cut it into bite-sized cubes, ensuring they are large enough to skewer.

Pick Fresh Mint Leaves:

Wash and pick fresh mint leaves from the stems. Choose smaller leaves for easy threading.

Slice Limes:

Slice limes into thin rounds. You can cut them in half or quarters for a more manageable size.

Assemble Skewers:

Thread the watermelon cubes, fresh mint leaves, and lime rounds onto the wooden or bamboo skewers in a visually appealing pattern. Alternate the ingredients for a colorful presentation.

Arrange on a Platter:

Place the assembled Infused Watermelon Skewers on a serving platter.

Chill (Optional):

If not serving immediately, you can chill the skewers in the refrigerator for about 30 minutes for a refreshing and cool snack.

Serve and Enjoy:

Serve the Infused Watermelon Skewers at room temperature or chilled. Enjoy this hydrating and flavorful treat.

Tips:

• Experiment with other complementary fruits like berries or cucumber slices.

• Drizzle a touch of honey or balsamic glaze for added sweetness or acidity.

• Make the skewers more festive by using different shapes of watermelon using cookie cutters.

Nutrition Information (per serving):

- Calories: 30
- Protein: 0g
- Carbohydrates: 8g
- Fat: 0g
- Saturated Fat: 0g
- Cholesterol: 0mg
- Sodium: 0mg
- Fiber: 1g
- Sugar: 6g

HIBISCUS AND BERRY SORBET

Refreshing Sorbet Description:

Hibiscus and Berry Sorbet is a vibrant and refreshing frozen dessert that combines the floral notes of hibiscus with the sweet and tart flavors of mixed berries. This sorbet is visually stunning and a delightful way to cool down on hot days. Enjoy the burst of fruity goodness in every spoonful.

Ingredients:

• 1 cup dried hibiscus flowers

• 2 cups boiling Water

• 2 cups mixed berries (strawberries, blueberries, raspberries)

• 1/2 cup granulated sugar (adjust to taste)

• One tablespoon of fresh lemon juice

Instructions:

Steep Hibiscus Tea:

In a heatproof bowl, pour boiling water water over dried hibiscus flowers. Let it steep for about 15-20 minutes, allowing the water to absorb the hibiscus flavor. Strain the hibiscus tea and let it cool.

Blend Berries:

In a blender, combine the mixed berries and blend until smooth.

Mix Hibiscus Tea and Berry Puree:

In a large bowl, mix the hibiscus tea with the berry puree. Stir well to combine.

Add Sugar and Lemon Juice:

Add granulated sugar to the berry-hibiscus mixture, adjusting the sweetness to your liking. Stir in fresh lemon juice for a hint of acidity.

Taste and Adjust:

Taste the sorbet mixture and adjust the sugar and lemon juice as needed. The flavors should be vibrant and balanced.

Chill the Mixture:

Place the sorbet mixture in the refrigerator to chill for at least 2 hours.

Freeze in Ice Cream Maker:

Transfer the chilled sorbet mixture to an ice cream maker and churn according to the manufacturer's instructions until it reaches a sorbet consistency.

Transfer to a Container:

Transfer the churned sorbet to a lidded container and freeze for an additional 4 hours or until firm.

Serve and Enjoy:

Scoop the Hibiscus and Berry Sorbet into bowls or cones. Garnish with fresh berries or mint leaves if desired. Enjoy the calm and fruity bliss!

Tips:

• If you don't have an ice cream maker, pour the chilled mixture into a shallow dish, freeze for 2 hours, then stir with a fork every 30 minutes until firm.

• Experiment with other berries like blackberries or cherries for a unique flavor profile.

• Garnish with a hibiscus flower for an extra touch of elegance.

Nutrition Information (per serving):

• Calories: 120

• Protein: 1g

• Carbohydrates: 30g

• Fat: 0g

• Saturated Fat: 0g

• Cholesterol: 0mg

• Sodium: 5mg

• Fiber: 5g

• Sugar: 24g

CONCLUSION

In conclusion, Mast Cell Activation Syndrome (MCAS) represents a multifaceted challenge characterized by the dysregulated activity of mast cells and the subsequent release of inflammatory mediators that can manifest in a diverse array of symptoms affecting various organ systems. The journey to managing MCAS involves a comprehensive approach, and in recent years, the role of diet has emerged as a promising avenue for symptom control and improved quality of life.

The adoption of a histamine-restricted diet tailored to individual sensitivities has shown promise in minimizing triggers and mitigating symptoms associated with MCAS. The meticulous identification of trigger foods through collaboration with healthcare professionals, such as allergists and dietitians, allows for a nuanced and personalized dietary strategy. Additionally, exploring an anti-inflammatory diet underscores the potential benefits of mitigating overall inflammation in the body, potentially curbing the hyperactivity of mast cells.

However, it is essential to recognize that the landscape of MCAS and its management is continually evolving. While dietary modifications offer valuable tools in symptom management, they are just one facet of a comprehensive treatment plan. Medications, lifestyle adjustments, and ongoing medical supervision are integral to managing MCAS effectively.

As our understanding of MCAS deepens and research progresses, integrating dietary considerations into personalized treatment plans holds promise for refining therapeutic strategies. The collaboration between patients and healthcare professionals remains pivotal, ensuring that dietary modifications are not only practical but also safe and sustainable.

In the face of the complex nature of MCAS, ongoing research, increased awareness, and a holistic approach to patient care are essential. By continuing to explore the interplay between diet and mast cell activity, we may uncover new insights that contribute to more effective, tailored interventions for individuals navigating the challenges posed by Mast Cell Activation Syndrome.